My
Aching
Back!

My Aching Back!

by **Nancy C. Selby**

Illustrations by Ann Sury

Technical consultants:
David F. Fardon, M.D.
David K. Selby, M.D.

✿ THE BODY PRESS

Published by The Body Press
A division of Price Stern Sloan, Inc.
360 North La Cienega Boulevard
Los Angeles, CA 90048

10 9 8 7 6 5 4 3 2 1
Manufactured in the United States of America

Library of Congress Cataloging-in-Publication Data
Selby, Nancy C.
    My aching back!

    Includes index.
    1. Backache—Popular works. 2. Human mechanics.
3. Physical fitness I. Title.
RD771.B217S45   1988   617'.56   88-7610
ISBN 0-89586-705-2

ACKNOWLEDGMENTS

Every author has acknowledgments, but I have never appreciated the importance of those until I embarked on this project!

The first vote of appreciation has to go to the patients and friends who found the information from the Spine Education Center's Back School beneficial enough to encourage me to share it.

Roses go to my staff, which was more patient than the law should allow. They stayed late, went in early, covered for me when I disappeared to the word processor, and generally tolerated the erratic and frantic behavior of "the Author."

Then there are those whose efforts will never be adequately repaid, but who will be forever appreciated: Raquel Lopez, P.T., who became the technical advisor for the entire book and still managed to run the Back School without missing a beat; Beth Melton for all the proofing time in the midst of industrial training commitments; Gwen Smith for the typing and retyping while answering the phone; Ann Sury for meeting every deadline with her wonderful illustrations; and Susie Matthews for the honest feedback from a non-medical viewpoint.

Last, but never least, accolades go to my husband, Dave. Without his input, encouragement and support, none of it would have happened. May he never have to cook that much again!

Dedicated to the girls in my life:
Pam, Kathy, Susie, Betsy, Lorry, and Selby Elizabeth

CONTENTS

▼

Chapter 1
Your Spine: How Does It Work?.......... page 1

Chapter 2
Common Causes Of Back Pain: What's
Happening in Your Life Now? .... page 13

Chapter 3
Principles of Body Mechanics: Learning
"Ouch-Free" Movement................................. page 31

Chapter 4
Customized Body Mechanics: Safe
Activities for Work, Home and Play................. page 51

Chapter 5
Do I Have To? Exercises for the Back-Pain
Sufferer .... page 103

Chapter 6
Just In Case: First Aid and Home
Treatment.. page 137

Glossary .... page 157

Index .... page 163

PREFACE

One afternoon in the mid-1970s, while working through a busy office in my practice of orthopedic surgery, I came across a patient who was not responding to my treatment. I had given him physical therapy and medicine for his low-back pain, but none of this seemed to have helped substantially. As we finished discussing his case, his last question was, "What are you going to do now?"

Because the patient had no identifiable cause for his pain, I had very little more to offer him in the way of treatment. He was overweight, out of shape, and unable to return to normal activities. Was it totally my responsibility to take care of this individual? If he would agree to accept some responsibility for his life, what could he do to treat himself? What could he and I work out? I estimated that it was going to take several hours to sufficiently explain all of the things he should be doing to promote his own health care. It was not a practical solution, so a moment was lost. Neither one of us were very satisfied with the outcome of that encounter.

A short time later I read in several medical journals about successful patient education programs for persons with diabetes and hemophilia. It seemed that education could substantially decrease doctor visits and reduce general expense for these patients. With education, these patients could and were willing to assume some responsibility for their own health care.

About the same time a physical therapist and an orthopedic surgeon in Goteborg, Sweden, developed an educational program for individuals who had sustained back injuries. They prepared a sound/slide presentation showing pretty Swedish models exercising and using proper body mechanics. The content was good, but the presentation was not very applicable for a group of patients in north central Texas.

It was at that point that my wife, Nancy, intervened saying, "I think I can design a more appropriate program to explain low back pain than that tape." With a background in education and communication, she assimilated the information and redesigned the format to fit a varied patient population. The vocabulary was changed from scientific, medical jargon to simple understandable language. Thus the Spine Education Center was born. Unknowingly, she had just started a full-time job with a professional commitment that continues to this time.

Nancy believes that education should be fun as well as instructive. I think this is reflected in her Back School, and you will find that in this book. She has become an expert in low back care and has the ability to express this in terms we can all appreciate. I am hopeful that this book can be as helpful to you, the reader, as the Back School is to the patients in my practice. Even better, I am hopeful that you read this book before your pain gets so bad that you have to see a doctor. It may save you suffering and money.

I know that Nancy has put in a lot of time and effort to produce a book that is easy to read and easy to apply. The only other ingredient needed is a reader willing to assume the responsibility for his or her own back care. After all, only the back owner lives with his back 24 hours a day, and only the back owner completely controls the activities and forces on the back. So read carefully. The back you save may be your own.

David K. Selby, M.D.

AUTHOR'S NOTE

No one writes a book without a good reason, and mine was the positive patient response to information—both verbal and written—presented in the Spine Education Center's Back School.

For the last eight years I have worked with employers and employees who are trying to reduce back injuries and resulting back pain. Those experiences have made me realize that everyone needs this information, because back pain is not merely an occupational hazard.

In the Back School, we try to allay fears associated with back pain. Now the Back School comes to the printed page. I hope this book not only calms your fears, but shows you how you can live comfortably with back pain—or banish it from your life.

N.S.

My
Aching
Back!

1

▼

Your Spine:
How Does It Work?

Your back's gone out. Again. The last time it happened, you were in bed for a week. You are supposed to leave for the Grand Canyon with the kids tomorrow. Now what? Do you cancel the trip, go to the emergency room and see if they will give you drugs, or do you just grit your teeth and hope it will go away overnight? All you did was lean over to pick up that pencil that dropped to the floor from your desk! How could anything that simple cause so much trouble?

The circumstances may vary, but the frustrations remain the same. Back pain, no matter when or where it occurs, is a scary and exasperating experience.

This book will teach you some techniques to make you more comfortable if you have back pain. Even more important, it will help you avoid back pain in the first place. You will be able to continue doing all the things you like to do. You will simply learn to do them more easily, better and with less back pain—or maybe no pain at all.

We are going to cover many activities that you do every day at work and at home. We are also going to give you suggestions for doing recreational activities painlessly by using your body to greatest advantage and putting the least amount of pressure on your back. Body awareness and understanding will give you the control that is essential to eliminate pain and aggravation from back and neck problems.

One reason back pain is so frustrating is because you cannot see what is happening. If you sprain your ankle, you can watch it swell and turn black-and-blue. A doctor can explain what is happening, when you will recover, and

▼

what first aid you should use. As he or she talks to you, your ankle provides visual proof that the recommendations are relevant to the injury. You may hurt physically, but you don't feel much emotional distress because you know it is only a matter of time before you return to activities you enjoyed before the sprain. The same is true with a knee, elbow or hand injury.

However, when you have a back injury or backache, communication is difficult because you cannot see or touch the injured area. Even if you look at your back in a mirror, you can't see what is happening to your spine. Unless your back has received a direct blow, it will not swell or turn black-and-blue. Therefore, it is difficult to comprehend the problems associated with back pain unless you have a basic understanding of the spine. You don't need to become an expert, but the following short anatomy lesson should be helpful.

Think of the spine as a tall, skinny building—the Eiffel Tower, perhaps. (Figure 1) If you ever played with an erector set as a kid, you know that the foundation had to be sturdy enough to support the construction. The lower, or lumbar, portion of the spine is the foundation. It is also the part of the spine that gets the most abuse, because your upper torso rests on the lumbar spine. About 70% of your weight is in your upper body. The spine narrows between the hips and the head because it does not have to support as much weight.

The back, like any structure, has parts that hold it together. The vertebrae link together to form the spine; they are the scaffolding of the back and neck.

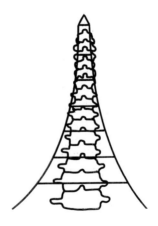

Figure 1
The spine resembles the Eiffel Tower.

Your spine has two basic functions. The first is support. The *vertebrae*, together with the muscles and ligaments that surround them, provide the support system. (Figure 2) Your spine enables you to stand, walk and move easily with your head in an upright position. The spine keeps you from looking like Raggedy Andy.

The second function of the spine is to protect the spinal cord, just as the covering on an electrical cord protects the wires inside. The spinal cord, an extension of your brain, runs through the middle of the spine. It is protected by the column of bone, or vertebrae.

Your spine has five anatomical sections: cervical spine, thoracic spine, lumbar spine, sacrum, and tailbone (coccyx). (Figure 3) If you stand sideways and look in a mirror, you will see that your back forms an "S" shape. The top of the "S" is your neck, or *cervical spine*, composed of seven vertebrae. Your middle spine is the *thoracic spine;* it has twelve vertebrae. The next five vertebrae make up your lower back, which is the *lumbar spine*. These 24 mobile vertebrae rest on a base composed of the *sacrum* and *tailbone (coccyx)*. The sacrum is made up of five vertebrae that are attached to each other. The tailbone is the last four vertebrae, which are also attached to each other. Although we will be concerned primarily with your lumbar spine, we will also touch upon the cervical spine and thoracic spine. The sacrum and tailbone are important, but they do not affect the way you feel as do the other sections of the spine.

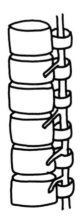

Figure 2
The vertebrae are in a column.

The spine has one additional function—motion—that is usually not incorporated into a building's design (unless it is earthquake-proofed). The spine's motion is carefully controlled at each vertebra by muscles and ligaments. If you compared the spine to the Eiffel Tower, the motion would occur at each landing. (Figures 4, 5)

Because protection of the spinal cord is critical, the vertebrae form an arch called the *lamina* that keeps the cord from being exposed. However, instead of running from the bottom of the neck to the tailbone in one column, this arch is divided into 24 active segments that allow you to bend over to tie your shoes, or turn your body to play golf or tennis. (Figure 6)

Each of these 24 segments has a similar structure: two joints, called *facet joints,* with an intervertebral disc in the middle. The discs are ingeniously

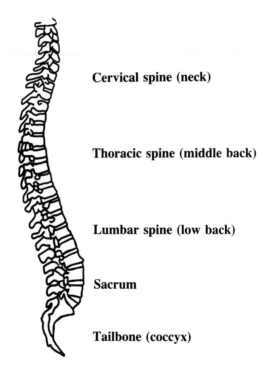

Cervical spine (neck)

Thoracic spine (middle back)

Lumbar spine (low back)

Sacrum

Tailbone (coccyx)

Figure 3
5 Sections of Spine

designed structures that have dual functions. They are the bending points in this large column of support, and they also cushion the spine against force. The intervertebral discs are the "shock absorbers" of your body, much like the shock absorbers in your car. (Figure 7)

Now that you have an overview of the spine and its basic parts, let's look at how it works and why it reacts the way it does. Each of the three different sections of the spine—cervical, thoracic and lumbar—is responsible for different functions.

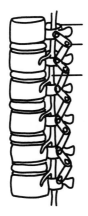

Figure 4

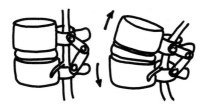

Figure 5
Motion occurs at each joint.

The cervical spine holds and stabilizes the head. Its joints are narrow and allow for rotational movement. The vertebrae support the head when you rotate it from side to side to say "no," move it up and down to say "yes," or tilt it to say "maybe." The cervical vertebrae are small and thin and house the vertebral artery. This important artery carries some of the blood supply to the brain.

Although the neck only has to hold up the head, it can cause difficulty when it is not cared for properly. Later you will learn exercises that reduce the stress in the neck area. These are particularly helpful if you spend a lot of time at a desk, on the telephone, or in front of a typewriter or computer.

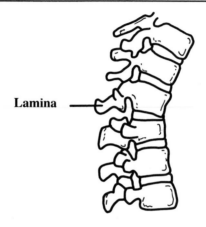

Lamina

Figure 6
Segmentations of lamina allow bending.

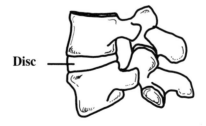

Disc

Figure 7
Discs are shock absorbers.

The thoracic spine supports your chest area. This is where the twelve ribs attach. The vertebrae in this area are bigger than the vertebrae in your neck. They must support the weight of your neck, shoulders, arms and hands. The thoracic spine allows you to move to turn your shoulders. If you are a golfer or a tennis player, you can appreciate how important this part of your spine is. Even though the joints that make up the thoracic spine are larger, some rotation can occur in your middle back.

The lumbar spine forms the bottom of the "S" curve that you observed when you looked in the mirror. Most of your body weight is supported by these last five vertebrae. As you might guess, the vertebrae in the lumbar spine are significantly larger so they can support your upper body. However, the joints between these larger vertebrae cannot rotate easily. This makes your lumbar spine particularly vulnerable to rotational or twisting injuries.

The discs, which allow motion at the bending segments of the spine, have two parts. The tough outer layer is called the *anulus fibrosus*. This is the cylinder that contains the soft inner portion, the *nucleus pulposus*. The name is almost self-explanatory. Nucleus means center, and pulposus describes the soft or pulp-like material inside the disc. (Figure 8)

The spine is constructed to allow for motion behind each disc. Facet joints are the "hinges" that allow motion; they are small joints situated between the arches of bone (lamina). (Figure 9) Not only do they permit motion at each joint, they also limit the amount of motion and specify the direction of motion.

Vertebra —
Anulus fibrosus —
Nucleus pulposus —

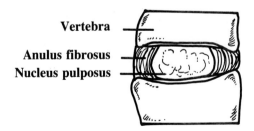

Figure 8
Two parts of the disc

Facet joints are not all the same size. At the top of the spine they are narrow and allow maximum motion. Toward the base of the spine they are wider and larger and designed to limit rotation. That is the reason you can rotate your head or turn around in your chair, but cannot twist your lumbar spine. The facet joints will not permit that much motion in the lower spine. Because rotation is difficult, the lumbar spine is more vulnerable to twisting incidents than the cervical or thoracic areas of the spine.

If discs are the shock absorbers in your body, why do they cause so much trouble? Like all other body parts, discs withstand a certain amount of wear and tear—no matter how well you take care of them. The wear and tear, or degeneration, is part of the aging process. We think about aging on the outside of our bodies, but not the inside. Disc degeneration represents the "gray hair and wrinkles" of the spine.

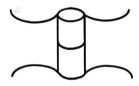

Figure 9
Facet joints are the hinges.

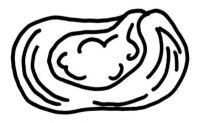

Figure 10
Bulging disc

▼

Although discs undergo a natural aging process, inappropriate use of the spine can accelerate disc degeneration. Unlike your car's shock absorbers, discs cannot be replaced if they wear out. Once discs have been abused, they cannot be regenerated. Therefore, using your discs as carefully as possible is critical to their longevity and your comfort.

Discs cushion the vibrations in the spine and keep the bones in the spine from rubbing together. If the disc is abused, it is likely to bulge. (Figure 10) It is easy to think about the disc as a jelly donut. If you squeeze too hard on a jelly donut, the jelly is going to squirt out at the weakest point. If you abuse the disc, the nucleus pulposus is going to rupture, or herniate, at the weakest point. (Figure 11) The terms "rupture" and "herniate" are used interchangeably in the medical community. Ruptured or herniated disc is the most common reason for back surgery.

The discs give the spine its height. You are tallest at about age 20; then you begin to shorten just a little each year as your discs age and lose some of their resiliency and water content. Fortunately, it is a slow process, but we all know individuals—grandparents, parents, elderly friends—who have "shrunk before our eyes." When the astronauts came back from the moon, they were a little taller than they were when they left; in outer space, gravity did not exert force on their discs, allowing their discs to expand. Because you can't see your discs, it is hard to remember the important role they play in the way you look and feel.

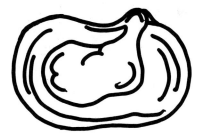

Figure 11
Herniated or ruptured disc

▼

Ligaments are the "guy wires" of the spine. They allow motion to occur, but only limited amounts. Each vertebra is connected to the next by ligaments, which are strong and tight. The ligaments that run the length of the spine in front and back also protect the discs and prevent them from moving backward or forward.

Muscles are the motors of the spine, as they are throughout the body. Because of their location and the way they connect to the bones and ligaments of the back, they provide the power to move the spine.

Muscles give the spine stability, flexibility, and the ability to withstand great loads. This includes such activities as lifting, carrying, pushing and pulling. Muscles also absorb the energy of sudden stresses, protecting the bones and ligaments from injury. Unfortunately, muscles are not maintenance-free. Without exercise and continual use, muscles become weak and cease to function efficiently.

Last—but hardly least—are the nerves. Nerves are the body's communication system, the "telephone wires" of the building. The spinal cord relays messages back and forth between the nerves and the brain. (Figure 12) The nerves carry those messages to and from muscles, skin, and other sensory organs.

Nerves come off the spinal cord as projections called *nerve roots*. The nerves from the cervical spine carry messages to the muscles to give you

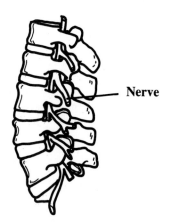

Figure 12
Nerves take messages to the brain.

▼

movement or from the skin to indicate sensations in the neck, shoulders, arms and hands. The thoracic nerves carry messages to the chest and the middle part of the back. The lumbar nerves carry messages to the lower back, pelvis, stomach, groin, legs and feet. For that reason, leg and hip disorders are frequently diagnosed as lumbar spine problems rather than extremity-related conditions.

The *sciatic nerve* is a significant messenger in warning of a back problem. The sciatic nerve is formed from multiple nerve roots of the lumbar spine. It sends signals down the leg to control the muscles, and up the leg to provide sensation. It is frequently involved in problems concerning the lumbar spine, because it originates there. Many problems in the low back affect the sciatic nerve and are reflected by pain down the leg, sensory change, or even muscle weakness.

The nerves extend from the spinal cord out of the spine through canals in the vertebrae. A nerve can become compressed or pinched when this opening gets too small from bone buildup, or when the disc wears out. Nerves can also become compressed if a disc bulges or ruptures, and nucleus pulposus presses against one of the lumbar nerves. Compressed nerves can cause pain and numbness in every part of the body, but these are particularly common in the lumbar spine region. The communication system works instantly—usually with pain—when one of these nerves, or "telephone wires," is involved.

So these are the basic components, or building blocks, of the spine. The spine is sturdy and flexible. It protects the spinal cord and will last a lifetime with adequate care and maintenance. If abused, however, it can cause serious problems and haunting pain.

Only one person can take care of your back: you, the back owner. Listening for the signals that warn of problems is necessary if you are to avoid permanent damage. Consider your options as we discuss common reasons for back pain and first-aid techniques, and introduce ways you can modify your activities. You do have options!

Taking care of your back is a little like dental hygiene. Both cavities and back pain can be kept to a minimum, but it takes some effort. There is nothing difficult about using a toothbrush or dental floss, but it requires dedication to good health habits. Changing the way you treat your back isn't going to be difficult either. The hardest part is making the commitment to use what you learn. However, a pain-free life is worth the effort. ▼

▼

Common Causes
of Back Pain:

What's Happening in Your Life Now?

There are many reasons for back pain. It can be caused by lifestyle, aging, disease or injury. Some types of pain, such as that caused by overexertion, are very common. Approximately 60 percent of industrial injuries are from overexertion. Other types, such as congenital deformities, are very rare.

Understanding the most common problems and diagnoses will help you know what to expect and how to avoid future recurrences of pain. For example, did you know that once a person has had an injury, he or she is four times more likely to have a second one? So if you have already experienced the dreaded "down in your back," it may happen again!

The most frequent causes of back pain will be presented in alphabetical order: arthritis, emotional stress, exertion injuries, lifestyle changes, muscle spasm, obesity, osteoporosis, overload injuries, posture problems, predisposing conditions, and traumatic occurrences, including ruptured discs. As a group, these problems cause back and/or neck pain for a large percentage of the population. However, the frequency with which these problems occur does not mean that solutions to them are simple.

It is impossible to determine which problem is most serious. If *you* are experiencing back pain, it is serious, no matter what its medical cause. If you understand the cause of your pain, you can take all the appropriate measures that will speed healing and keep "down time" to a minimum. In later chapters you will learn how to modify daily activities and do exercises that relate to your specific pain-producing experiences.

Now let me give you some surprising statistics. Seventy percent of all back pain will go away in two to three weeks, no matter what is done. In six weeks,

90 percent of all back pain will disappear, regardless of treatment. And 98 percent of all back pain will disappear in three months if the person and the doctor do absolutely nothing! You may be skeptical of these figures, because statistics can be manipulated to indicate almost anything the writer wants to convey. However, these conclusions come from controlled studies done by spine specialists over many years. So the odds are in your favor that your back pain will disappear within two weeks to three months if you do nothing more than tolerate the inconvenience.

That's the good news. The bad news is that with each recurring incident, the chances for a serious problem increase dramatically, and the possibility for additional injuries also increases. How much time can you spend away from your job and your family? How much time are you willing to spend flat on your back at home or in the hospital. Are you prepared to suffer the consequences of back surgery? Probably not. Therefore, it is a good idea to recognize the factors that trigger your back or neck pain and do something about them before pain becomes a serious problem in your life.

ARTHRITIS

Ed was frustrated. He had bought the most expensive "orthopedic" mattress on the market, and he still had back and neck pain. The pain seemed to diminish late in the day, but it was there every morning. He considered buying a water bed, but his bank account was in no condition for more expensive mistakes.

Ed decided to see his doctor before he made the purchase. Unfortunately, his pain wasn't caused by the mattress, and a water bed wouldn't help. Ed had arthritis.

Did you ever spend time worrying about getting arthritis? Of course not. But you have known about it since you were a child, because adults always talked about having arthritis in their knees, fingers and other joints. You thought it only happened when people got old. Yet here you are, young, and you have arthritis—it makes you feel old. Don't despair. It may not be as bad as you think.

The term "arthritis" ordinarily does not refer to a disease; it means inflammation of a joint. There are two types of arthritis. The most common type is caused by degenerative wear-and-tear on the joints—the aging process. Have you ever noticed how often older people have swollen knuckles? This is a symptom of arthritis and is the result of many years of use.

The second type of arthritis is caused by disease—whether it be rheumatoid arthritis or some other aggressive joint disease. Arthritic disease in the lumbar spine is rare. Most people who have a diagnosis of arthritis of the spine are experiencing the degenerative process, which is a condition caused by aging.

The natural aging of the facet joints in the back of your spine or the aging of the discs in the front is a common reason for low back pain. The lining around the joint can also become inflamed and cause back pain. Degenerative changes will cause a loss of water content in the discs and will affect the amount of motion available in the spine. The narrowing of the discs, the wearing down of the facet joints and the inflammation of the lining around the joints can result in arthritis-like changes.

Now that you have heard the bad news, it is time to look on the bright side. While arthritis in the low back is a common diagnosis and can cause discomfort, it is important to remember that it is a process of wear and tear. Just because your back is affected is not to imply that you will have serious problems in other joints.

Anti-inflammatory medication will usually control the discomfort, and modifying your daily activities will allow you to do anything you want to do. These tasks and options will be discussed in Chapter 3. Specific exercises such as swimming will also be recommended in Chapter 5.

If you are diagnosed as having some other type of arthritis, your physician will prescribe special medication and warn you of additional precautions you should take.

EMOTIONAL STRESS

Donna was late getting home because her boss insisted that she finish typing all the letters he had dictated after being out of town for five days. Her 16-year-old daughter was in the middle of a raging battle with her stepfather. Dinner had not been started, and the den was a disaster area, littered with pop cans and empty bags of chips. As she walked in, her daughter stomped out, yelling something about "not being fair." By the time Donna had cooked and cleaned up the kitchen and the mess, she was exhausted. In addition to the terrible day, she had a headache and her back hurt! (Figure 13)

Muscles can do only one thing well, and that is contract. Emotional stress contributes to back and neck pain because muscles react quickly to their environment. You may be using excellent body mechanics, but stress may be controlling your life and causing you discomfort. Progressive relaxation exercises may help when things get tense. These will be presented in detail in Chapter 6.

EXERTION INJURIES

Sam was sitting at his desk going over the proposed budget for the year and suddenly noticed his back was aching. He squirmed a few times and then settled back to complete the task he had been working on for two weeks. If the budget was not exact, he might not be able to implement all of his great ideas, so he had spent all day and half of each night carefully going over each figure. He had even taken the project home. The family had been pretty tolerant of his neglect. The report was due today, and the weekend was here, so he could make up for all of the time he had not spent with Randy, Seth and Alice.

Driving home, Sam let out a sigh of relief. He had done the best he could. Now it was up to his boss to decide if the funding would be available. "I'll change my clothes, get the lawn mowed in a hurry and maybe try jogging a couple of miles. I haven't done anything physical for so long! I guess I ought to throw the ball with the kids, too. Tomorrow I'll get the garage cleaned out. We have accumulated a lot of junk since we moved in, and I have been promising to do that for six months."

Sam had a nagging back pain; it was not serious, but noticeable. As he got out of his suit, he noticed his back was bothering him. He attributed it to inactivity, which was probably true.

Out in the yard, he tackled the first job on his list. The lawn wasn't large and the mower was powered, but he had to lean over to clip around the trees and the edge of the sidewalk. "Why don't I spend the money and buy an automatic edger? I'll do that next week!" he said to himself for the fiftieth time.

With the lawn under control and a little daylight left, he threw the football to the boys a few times. Then he decided to jog a quick mile to soothe his conscience because he had had no real exercise in several weeks. His back still

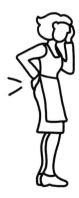

Figure 13
Emotional stress can cause back pain.

ached, but it wasn't too bad, and a hot shower seemed to help. After dinner, he stretched out on the couch to watch TV and placed the heating pad behind him. It sure felt good.

Sam could hardly get out of bed the next morning. The nagging backache had turned into real aggravation! Back to the couch and the heating pad—the garage could wait one more week. But the boys couldn't. They had tryouts for the football team on Monday, and they needed to practice with "the expert." So there went Sam, out to the park, throwing and running. The pain was there—but tolerable—and practice with the boys was important. Before he realized it, they'd practiced for several hours. (Figure 14)

He felt awful on Sunday morning and could barely creep around the house. Sam considered a trip to the local minor emergency clinic but decided that he really "hadn't done anything that should cause any serious damage." Resting all day would probably cure the problem. Back to the heating pad!

His back still hurt badly on Monday morning, but he had an important meeting on the budget proposal. He struggled to the shower, emerged feeling a little better, and drove 40 minutes to the office. When he got to his desk and reached into the bottom file drawer for the reports—bam! wham!—he felt excruciating pain! Sam had just experienced an exertion injury.

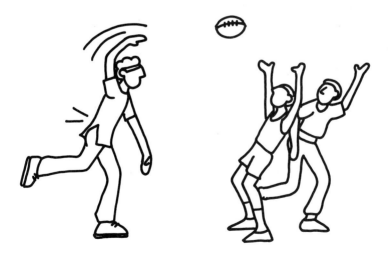

Figure 14
The weekend athlete is a back-pain candidate.

It may comfort Sam to know that almost all back pain disappears eventually. However, those weeks of discomfort and disability could have been avoided entirely with a little preplanning. Sam forgot that the activities he wanted to do were athletic in nature, and his body had been used to sitting, not moving. You can't surprise your muscles and not expect them to react. Muscles can react rather violently and trigger pain.

Because Sam has a desk job, he might not be off from work for long. If he were a truck driver, welder or furniture mover, he might be off the job for six weeks. That is a long time to be out of work when you are the breadwinner.

LIFESTYLE CHANGES

Susie was always active. In fact, she almost drove her parents crazy because she was involved with so many extracurricular activities as a teen. Swimming, gymnastics, dancing and cheerleading were her life during junior high and high school. She even continued with an aerobics class during college. When she graduated, she moved to Chicago and took a job with a big insurance agency, processing accounts.

Susie was busy, but she managed to get to the health spa at least three times a week and walk to the office whenever the weather permitted. After she and Mark married, however, the exercise routine became more difficult. Something always interfered with her exercise time. Once they moved to the suburbs and she became pregnant, exercise seemed impossible.

Now 32, Susie is miserable! Her back hurts all the time. She has gained 14 pounds since she married. Keeping up with a six-year-old and a two-year-old is exhausting, and she spends most days cleaning, cooking or running errands in her car. (Figure 15)

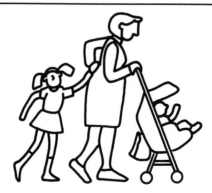

Figure 15
Lifestyle changes can reduce muscle tone.

▼

Lifestyle changes have contributed to Susie's back-pain problem. Although she is very busy, the activities are not the kind that will protect her back from injury. Susie does not consider herself a sedentary person, but from the standpoint of physical conditioning, flexibility and muscle strength, she might as well be.

Lifestyle changes creep up on you. They generally signify a change that decreases physical fitness, increases weight, and sometimes modifies your posture. If you have been active and are suddenly relegated to a desk job, you may find those abdominal and quadriceps (thigh) muscles deteriorating very quickly. They can no longer give your spine the kind of support they did in the past.

Do you remember when you first started feeling that nagging backache? Could it be from a change in your lifestyle? You may have to make some *conscious* changes so you can get rid of your back pain. Being busy does not mean being physically fit.

MUSCLE SPASM

Muscles! They seem to affect everything we do, and they are always cramping or tightening! There is a reason for that. Muscles can only "do" two things. They can contract and constrict, or they can relax; but they can't relax without help, so what they do best is tighten. Muscle spasm is the most common reason for back pain. If it has ever happened to you, you know how uncomfortable and painful it can be.

The muscles around the spine add protection. If you overexert those muscles, the messages to the brain say, "contract, contract, contract." Because muscles are designed to protect, they set off an alarm when they are mistreated, and a back injury without muscle involvement is rare. However, muscles that are warmed up, flexible, and strong do not react as violently when a strange or unusual situation occurs.

Professional athletes know that to decrease their chances of injury, stretching and strengthening their muscles before an event is very important. A professional weightlifter would be foolish if he did not work up to his maximum lift gradually. Yet, some people think they can lean over and lift groceries or suitcases out of the trunk of the car just after they have been sitting for 30 minutes, stuck in traffic. Is it any wonder they end up with back pain and severe muscle spasm? Of course not. It is the only reaction muscles can have to lack of consideration! Fortunately, some first-aid techniques for muscle spasm are very effective; these will be discussed in Chapter 6.

Our alarm system triggers pain, which is our indicator that we are not taking good care of our backs. Listen to the messages from those muscles.

▼

OBESITY

Donald is 5'9" and weighs 240 pounds. He is a truck driver with constant back pain. His doctor has X-rayed his spine and found nothing wrong. He has seen a chiropractor off and on for the past two years, has been to the physical therapist, has taken muscle relaxants and anti-inflammatory medications, and nothing has helped. His back still hurts!

Does Donald's back hurt because he is overweight, or does it hurt because he is so deconditioned that he cannot perform the exercises and body-mechanics positions that would protect his back and reduce the stress? Does obesity by itself cause back pain? The experts say no. However, they have concluded that a person who is overweight is unable to recover from a bout of back pain as quickly as someone who is in fairly good physical condition.

It is a difficult problem to address. If obesity does not cause back pain, it certainly contributes to the discomfort level. The obese individual may have weak muscles, leaving the spine vulnerable and unprotected. Excess body weight also puts more pressure on the lumbar spine, joints and discs. While obesity does not seem to increase the incidence of back pain, it does affect one's ability to respond to treatment. Therefore, a serious diet and a physical conditioning program may be the only solution to Donald's constant pain.

OSTEOPOROSIS

Have you seen Elizabeth lately? She is beginning to get round-shouldered, and there is something wrong with her. She is only 59 years old, but lately she

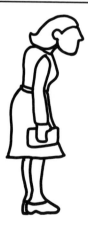

Figure 16
Osteoporosis

looks 70! She started looking old after she fell last winter and broke her wrist. Elizabeth had always been so cute and tiny. Her friends envied her blonde hair, blue eyes and size-6 figure, but she doesn't look good now.

Elizabeth has osteoporosis. The word means brittle bones, and Elizabeth's bones are beginning to look a little bit like Swiss cheese. That's why she broke her wrist. If the disease process continues, she is going to have fractures of the spine. In fact, she has probably already started the process, because her shoulders are beginning to stoop. (Figure 16) Poor Elizabeth! No one warned her in time about that early hysterectomy and the lack of estrogen in her body. Her osteoporosis could have been prevented.

Osteoporosis is a disease most commonly found in post-menopausal women. Fortunately, it is also a disease that can be prevented if you understand the causes and are aware of the potential problems and situations that cause osteoporosis. Who is a candidate for osteoporosis? Women are four times more susceptible than men. Women who are fair-haired, fair-skinned, of small bone structure, and from Northern European descent are more prone to this disease than those who are dark-skinned, larger-boned and of southern European or African heritage. Oriental women are also high-risk candidates. Due to genetic factors, women with family members who have or had osteoporosis also are more susceptible.

Because the disease causes brittle bones and loss of bone density, it contributes to broken hips, fractured limbs and the loss of height that so often occur in older people. Years ago, osteoporosis was not a great concern, because few people lived long enough for it to become a problem. However, in 1987, the average life expectancy for women is 84 years. If age 50 is used as the average age for menopause, it does not take a mathematician to figure out that women will be susceptible to bone-mass deterioration for 34 years. Women who have had surgical hysterectomies may be even more prone to the disease, particularly if the ovaries that produce hormones have been removed.

Estrogen is produced while the ovaries are active and protects against osteoporosis. Once the ovaries are inactive, either due to the natural aging process or surgical removal, estrogen replacement therapy may be prescribed. Although we don't know exactly why, estrogen helps reduce hot flashes, decreases anxiety and depression, preserves normal vaginal function and contributes greatly to maintaining bone density.

Early studies reported a link between estrogen and uterine cancer. However this has been refuted by leading gynecologists and researchers who support the studies showing that estrogen taken in appropriate dosages is safe. Progesterone is often prescribed with estrogen. When taken with estrogen, progesterone actually protects against uterine cancer. The dosage varies with the individual and can only be determined by a doctor. Hormone therapy following menopause can help a woman to maintain a hormone balance that keeps her comfortable and healthy for many years.

Calcium is currently being investigated to determine whether a particular dosage or type of supplement is better than another. The recommended daily dosage for maintaining healthy bone density is approximately 1500mg. This requirement can be met in two ways—through calcium supplements or a diet high in calcium. A combination of the two is probably the most sensible approach.

Dairy products are the best calcium source, and skim-milk products have a higher calcium content than whole-milk products. This is good news for those who are reluctant to drink milk or eat cheese because of the high caloric value of dairy products. Leafy green vegetables such as broccoli, spinach and kale are also good calcium sources. They can be prepared with cheese sauce to increase their calcium content and enhance flavor. Low-fat yogurt has become popular and is readily available almost everywhere in the U.S. and even overseas. To better acquaint yourself with the calcium content of food products, read food labels as you shop for groceries.

Another measure essential for the prevention of osteoporosis is weight-bearing exercise. Weight-bearing exercise includes walking, jogging, dancing, aerobics, tennis, golf, volleyball, racquetball, bowling, roller-skating and any other activities that exert positive force on the spine. Swimming and bicycling are not weight-bearing activities. Although they are excellent for increasing strength and lung capacity and are recommended for the average back-pain patient, they are not the best exercises for the osteoporosis patient.

Because osteoporosis is preventable, it is important that young women be informed about it and start thinking about calcium intake and weight-bearing exercise long before problems develop. Encourage your daughters to begin a physical fitness program at an early age and maintain healthy bone density throughout their lives.

Specific exercises for osteoporosis patients and for prevention of osteoporosis will be presented in Chapter 5. Walking techniques will also be discussed.

OVERLOAD

As the van pulled into the loading dock, Dennis knew he was facing a long, tough day. The boxes of samples weighed 57 pounds each, and they had to be stacked on pallets to be distributed to the manufacturer's representatives later in the week. Even though he had a hand truck available, he still had to

▼

physically pick up each carton, stack it on the dolly, push the loaded dolly to the warehouse and unload the cartons from the dolly to a pallet on the floor. It wouldn't have been as difficult if his helper were there, but Jim had called in sick that morning, and no one else was free at the moment to help him. Because there were so many containers, Dennis decided that the only way he could finish in time was to stack four or five boxes at a time and move them quickly.

He started at 7:30 a.m. and finished the job just before lunch. He noticed by late morning that his back was sore and getting worse with each load. Although he did not work on the dock after lunch, his back pain increased. By the middle of the afternoon the pain was intolerable. Dennis was used to handling heavy material and prided himself on being in excellent physical condition, but the loads had been too heavy. (Figure 17)

Dennis had some alternatives that probably would have protected him: he could have waited for a helper; used a better mechanical device such as a forklift; or loaded only one or two cartons at a time. Then the weight would have been tolerable.

The injury that Dennis experienced is a form of overexertion injury, but is compounded by the weight of the material. The spine can withstand only so much weight before it rebels. An overload injury can result in a ruptured or herniated disc, which may require surgery.

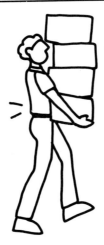

Figure 17
Overloading your spine can lead to a serious injury.

▼

The National Institute of Health and Safety estimates that most men in the U.S. can lift 36 pounds on a repetitive basis, and women can lift 28 pounds repetitively. That doesn't sound like much, but if you are having to pick up a load every minute—or even every five minutes—the spine is having to adjust to those loads very quickly. The body mechanics positions used are also critical in avoiding overload injuries. The position of the spine in relation to loads will be discussed in detail in Chapter 3.

Although Dennis was in good physical condition, the loads were excessive. Knowing your strength is important, but listening to your back is equally important. Dennis forgot that. Poor judgment may put Dennis in the hospital. Surgery and three to six months of recuperation are possible. Overloading your back in not worth the price.

POSTURE

Kathy took a job selling real estate after she finished school. Suddenly she had to dress up everyday, so Kathy began wearing high-heeled shoes. After years of wearing flat shoes or tennis shoes to school, the change in her activities was significant. She also started to have back pain. She thought it was because she was spending so many hours at her job, taking clients to look at houses, getting into and out of the car, etc. But most of her back pain was a result of a posture change. Wearing high-heeled shoes increased the curve in her low back, changed her posture, alarmed her muscles and triggered discomfort. (Figure 18) Kathy needs to recognize the benefit of using a two-inch or lower

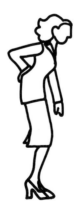

Figure 18
Posture affects your comfort level.

heel during her work day. Her posture will not be drastically affected, and she can save her very high heels for special occasions when she does not have to stand or walk for long periods of time.

Michael and Kathy finished school at the same time, and Michael went to work in a machine shop. Michael also began experiencing back pain, but his pain was related to standing on a concrete floor for eight hours a day in front of a machine. His back was used to sitting in a classroom. Once Michael discovered the cause of his back pain, he requested and received a rubber mat to stand on. He also used a railing next to his machine to prop up a foot while working. It was amazing how quickly his pain disappeared once he used good posture techniques and took pressure off his low back.

How do you sit? How do you stand? Has your posture changed as you have gotten older? Has your posture changed because you have a new chair or a new job? Do you use a computer instead of a typewriter? Do you stand on concrete or tile floors at work or in the kitchen? Your back and/or neck pain may be a result of a posture change.

Neck pain is often related to poor posture. If you have to sit all day looking at a computer screen, your head needs to be centered over your shoulders, and your back should be well-supported. Arm rests on the chair are also helpful.

If you arrive at home every evening with neck pain, shoulder discomfort and a headache, don't quit your job. Instead, rearrange your posture. You may have unknowingly become a head-thruster! If so, your muscles will react by

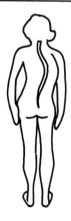

Figure 19
Scoliosis

tensing, because your neck is sensitive to good and bad positions. Specific exercises and body mechanics positions will be introduced later to correct aggravating neck problems.

Your posture can contribute to your discomfort or alleviate your pain. Listening to your back will give you the clues for positive posture.

PREDISPOSING CONDITIONS

Fourteen-year-old Betsy was really excited about the Valentine's Day dance. It would be her first "real" dance. She and her mom had shopped a long time for the perfect dress before they found it. The dress needed some alterations, and Betsy's mother had a difficult time getting the seams and hem straight. It was almost as if one hip were higher than the other. She thought nothing of it, though, because Betsy was changing so rapidly that it was almost impossible to keep her in clothes that fit. Several weeks after the dance, however, the school nurse called Betsy's parents. She recommended they take her to the doctor because she suspected that Betsy had scoliosis.

Predisposing conditions are those that are developmental or congenital. The following will give you a brief explanation of the most common of these, so you will better understand the terminology if it is used by your physician.

Conditions of structural abnormality have several characteristics. *Scoliosis,* better known as "curvature of the spine," is one of these. (Figure 19) It

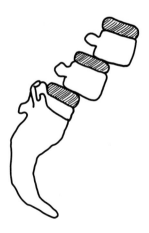

Figure 20
Spondylolisthesis

is more common in females than males. The seriousness of scoliosis is evaluated by degrees. A slight curvature of 10-15 degrees might not be bothersome, while a serious curvature of 60 degrees might require surgery and/or bracing. Scoliosis was a serious and relatively common problem a number of years ago, but has become controllable in recent times. Many elementary schools now provide scoliosis screening, so the problem is often recognized early when intervention is most effective. However, it is possible that a small degree of curve can increase in later life, can become painful and may require a medical evaluation by your doctor.

Spondylolisthesis affects approximately five percent of the population, and most of these individuals don't know they have it. The word is so long that the disease sounds frightening. (Figure 20) It means that the fifth lumbar vertebra has a forward displacement upon the sacrum, or less commonly, the fourth lumbar vertebra is on the fifth lumbar vertebra. The cause is a loss of bony continuity in the most narrow part of the arch between the lamina and facet joint. This can be diagnosed by X-ray. If it is severe, surgery to fuse the spine may be necessary to stabilize the spine. It is more common for an individual to go through life unaware of the abnormality.

Spina bifida means a forked or separated spine. The arches fail to form over the spinal cord of the developing fetus, leaving no protection between the spine and the cord. It is a serious abnormality in infants, but it can often be corrected surgically. Another term that is frequently used, *spina bifida occulta*, means a small separation of bone; it is not thought to be a painful, dangerous or unstable condition. If your doctor suddenly tells you that you have spina bifida, and you are totally unaware of any kind of abnormality, he is most likely talking about the latter deformity.

Other anatomical abnormalities occasionally show up on X-ray, such as four lumbar vertebrae instead of five, or six instead of five. Neither of these conditions causes problems. It is also possible for a person to have poorly formed vertebrae at birth, but this is rare.

All of these conditions are unusual, but may show up in later years. If you have been healthy all your life and thought that your spine was perfect, it may be a shock to discover that it is not. But even with some abnormalities, you can continue a normal life doing most of the activities you enjoy. The way you do those activities may require some modification, but the change will prevent problems later.

TRAUMATIC OCCURRENCES

Although accidental back injuries do occur, they are easily identifiable and actually more rare than back pain related to degeneration or overexertion. The most common injury is a compression fracture, which usually occurs as a result of a fall or some kind of trauma. Depending on the severity of the injury, it may cause discomfort and continual problems, and may require surgical intervention and stabilization.

RUPTURED DISC

Over the years, Tony had had several bouts of back pain. The first episode occurred while he was wind-surfing and struggling with the sail. The pain only lasted for a few days. The second time came after a car trip of several days. Again the pain disappeared in a few days. From then on, Tony had occasional bouts of back pain; each seemed to last a little longer than the last, but all eventually disappeared. One sunny afternoon on the golf course, Tony took a mighty swing at the ball. Suddenly, he felt pain down the back of his leg. His back hurt, too, but not as much as his leg. He had hip pain and a burning sensation down the side of his leg to his foot. This time the pain did not go away in a few days. Tony had ruptured a disc in his low back.

A ruptured or herniated disc is probably the most common, serious source of back pain. It can be a result of traumatic injury but is more often the result of degeneration. As mentioned earlier, the disc resembles a jelly donut. When the pressure becomes too great, the outer edges weaken and allow the jelly to squirt out. People with ruptured discs often complain of leg and hip pain

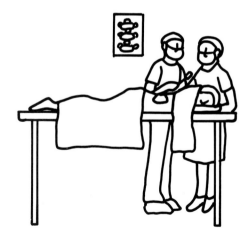

Figure 21
The solution to a ruptured disc may be surgery.

because the jelly-like material, or nucleus pulposus, touches or presses on nerves that send messages to the leg. A herniated disc also can cause tingling and pain in the foot. This is normally corrected by removing the disc material that affects the nerve. Although recovery from this surgery may require three weeks to three months, most people—depending on job and lifestyle—return to normal activities and are not restricted in any way. (Figure 21)

There are many possible causes of low back pain, but almost all can be controlled by some means. If you are aware of why you are uncomfortable, you can change what you do and how you do it to control the severity of your problem and minimize your discomfort. The next several chapters are devoted to constructive suggestions for avoiding back pain, regardless of the cause.

3

Principles of Body Mechanics:
Learning "Ouch-Free" Movement

Now that you understand how your spine works and some of the causes of back pain, you are ready for the next step on the road to a pain-free back. This part is fun and easy; you are going to become a participant rather than an observer.

You have heard the phrase "you can't teach an old dog new tricks," but you know that isn't true. If the reward is special, even a very old dog will give it his best shot. So don't think for a minute that you "can't" change. The tricks you are going to learn are body-mechanics modifications, and the reward is control of your back pain.

"What in the world is body mechanics?" you ask. *Body mechanics is your body's posture or position and its relationship to your activity or environment.* Unfortunately, most school systems do not offer courses in body mechanics. In fact, most of us learn habits at an early age that contribute to back pain in later life. Therefore, it is doubly beneficial for you to become a body-mechanics expert so you can share the information with your children.

Bill and Jesse each have jobs that require extensive travel by automobile and airplane. They are both in their early forties, successful, have full-sized luxury cars, belong to a health facility and pride themselves on being in good physical condition. Bill never has back pain. Jesse frequently complains about his back aching when he returns from one of his sales trips. What is the difference? To the unpracticed eye they look exactly the same. As sales representatives, they are handling product samples, driving long hours, carrying suitcases into and out of hotels and airport terminals and generally maintaining the same lifestyle. There is one major difference. Bill understands and practices good body mechanics, but Jesse doesn't. Once you are knowledgeable about body mechanics, we'll take you through a day in their lives and see if you can identify their differences.

If you have ever thought about body mechanics at all, you have probably thought about lifting. For years, proper lifting techniques have been taught in industry, with a goal of reducing back injuries. But it has not been effective. Back injuries continue to plague the work force. Unfortunately, the lifting training has usually consisted of a film that is totally irrelevant to the material being handled by the viewer. For example, if you have to move bulky metal valves, watching a model in a studio handle an eight-inch-square box is hardly pertinent.

Body-mechanics training includes lifting techniques, but it also includes daily activities such as sitting, standing, bending, turning, reaching, pushing, pulling and squatting. Every action you perform from the time you wake up in the morning until you wake up the next morning involves body mechanics. Hence, the use of good body mechanics needs to be an ongoing project. While poor lifting practices contribute to back problems, other body postures do too.

Body mechanics is related to how much pressure is placed on the lumbar discs in various positions. In the early 1970s, a study was done in Goteborg, Sweden, to determine how much intervertebral pressure an individual was actually placing on the low discs through various movements. The pressure was measured in kilograms and translated for Americans to pounds per square inch. This notable study has been the standard for spine specialists in the medical profession for the past 15 years. The numbers, which will be indicated as pounds per square inch, will be used here to show you which postures in your daily activities are uncomfortable for your low back and which are desirable. The larger the numbers, the higher the disc pressure.

Athletes tend to be in tune with their bodies. In other words, they know if everything is functioning normally, if a muscle is abused, if something is stressed or if they need to limber up before they start an event. They become so "body-aware" that they know what limits their muscles and ligaments will have under certain conditions. Although you may not be an athlete, you need to develop the same kind of awareness about your spine and your body.

If you learn to listen to your back, you will be able to tell when you are putting too much pressure on your lumbar discs. *Awareness is the key ingredient when you are trying to protect yourself.* Awareness provides you with positive and negative feedback, although it sometimes takes several hours in an undesirable position before your back reminds you that you aren't using appropriate body mechanics. By that time you may be in pain.

Your goal should be to develop such a high awareness level that you will know immediately whether something needs to be changed. This could mean changing something about your posture, your environment or both.

SITTING

Americans have a high incidence of back-pain episodes compared to people of other countries. One of the main reasons for this is that we have become a nation of sitters. Most people sit at their jobs, whether they are in an office or on an assembly line. They sit in their car going to and from work. They sit in front of the television set, sit to watch their kids play football, baseball or soccer, sit during piano lessons and dance recitals, and sit while they eat. They even sit when it might be better if they stood up. For example, a person with a desk job who frequently uses the telephone would eliminate much disc pressure if he or she stood while talking.

Did you realize that sitting puts a lot of pressure on the low-back discs, particularly if you sit in a slouched or slumped position? If you sit hunched over your desk or work area, it is possible that you're putting 200 lbs. of pressure per square inch on the lumbar discs. (Figure 22) If you sit in a slouched position while watching television, you are probably putting about 150 lbs. per square inch on those critical discs. (Figure 23) It may feel comfortable while you are engrossed in your favorite program, but it also may

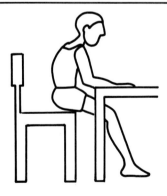

Figure 22
Sitting like this can put 200 lbs. of pressure per square inch on the lumbar discs.

be the body-mechanics position that causes you to wake up in the morning with a backache. That's the problem with bad body-mechanics positions. Unless you become an expert, you may not realize that the position you use in the afternoon may affect how you feel the next day or even the next week.

Have you ever taken a long car trip or plane ride? After several hours in that confined space, you begin to notice some back discomfort. Squirming may help a little but not enough to eliminate the nagging ache. The only thing that relieves the discomfort is getting out of the seat and moving around. The reason this makes you more comfortable is that you have listened to your back and are reducing the low-back pressure by standing up.

Body-mechanics positions almost always can be modified no matter what you are doing. Let's look at some ways you can change your sitting posture. If you sit with your knees higher than your hips, you decrease the disc pressure by as much as 50 percent. (Figure 24)

How do you sit? Have you looked at your chair recently? The chair may be fine, but you may be too short. You should be able to sit very comfortably with your feet flat on the floor without putting pressure on the back of your thighs. If this is not the case, place your feet on a small stool or on the rungs of your chair to take the pressure off your lumbar discs. This will make your back feel more comfortable, especially if you have to sit for many hours in one place. In Chapter 4, you will learn how to make this work for you whether you are in a car, a plane, on an assembly line or at your desk. You can even learn how to watch television for hours without hurting your lumbar discs.

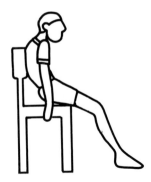

Figure 23
The "All-American slouch" can cause back pain because it puts
150 lbs. of pressure on the low-back discs.

STANDING

Have you ever noticed how chairs seem to disappear at big parties or receptions? There you are, in your best clothes, your highest high heels, trying to juggle a plate of food and a drink, and there is not a chair in sight. You try to

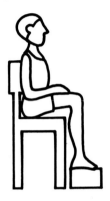

Figure 24
Sitting with your knees higher than your hips can reduce disc pressure. This is only 100 lbs. per square inch.

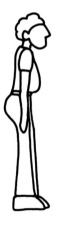

Figure 25
Standing at attention with your knees locked puts 200 lbs. of pressure on your low back and makes your back tired.

▼

pretend you are having a marvelous time with "your best foot forward," but your back hurts so much you want to scream. Instead, you grin and bear it and leave as soon as possible.

In anticipation of the next one of these extravaganzas you must attend, practice changing your standing habits now. Your new habits won't make a fun party out of a boring event, but they will make it more tolerable.

Remember how posture can affect the way your back feels? Standing with your knees locked can put as much as 200 lbs. of pressure per square inch on the low-back discs. (Figure 25) That is the same amount of pressure as sitting in a bent-forward position.

From the time you were small you were taught to "stand up straight, stand at attention, stand tall." But your instructors forgot to tell you what that was doing to your back. There are three natural curves in the spine, but those curves need an occasional rest. If you literally "put your best foot forward," you will decrease the amount of pressure on your back. This creates a *diagonal stance* and gives you a wide base of support, giving your back a rest. (Figure 26) Try standing at attention and placing your hand behind your back to feel the lumbar curve. Then move your feet into a diagonal stance. You should feel the curve in your low back flatten. Changing your standing posture

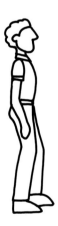

Figure 26
A diagonal stance with one foot in front of the other can reduce disc pressure by 50 percent.

▼

this way reduces the disc pressure to 100 lbs. per square inch. If you have to stand for any length of time, this makes a big difference. (Figure 27)

There are a couple of other modifications you can make to further protect yourself. You can tighten your abdominal muscles and tuck in your buttocks. Make sure you continue breathing while you do this! This technique is not an easy one to master unless you practice it everyday. This position, often called the "pelvic tilt," puts your spine in a neutral (non-stressful) plane. It is a body-mechanics technique you can use without being obvious. You can practice it while standing in line at the movies or standing around socializing with your friends. Tightening your abdominal muscles will also give your spine additional support from the front. Strong back muscles and abdominal muscles are necessary for adequate control.

If the diagonal stance feels strange, try putting a foot up on a stool or railing. This body-mechanics position is simply a variation of the same standing posture. Have you ever wondered how people can stand around for hours in a neighborhood pub and seem to be totally comfortable? They are comfortable because they have a foot propped up on the brass railing, which takes a great deal of pressure off the lower back. Using the diagonal stance with a foot propped up should be forever known as the "bar-resting position." (Figure 28) If you have not tried this standing position, you should. Look around for a

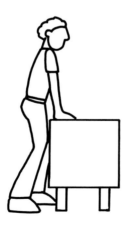

Figure 27
The diagonal stance will protect your back in many different situations.

place to put a foot up. If a railing isn't available, a low stool or a telephone book from a large city will provide the right height for a comfortable stance.

HANDLING LOADS

There are some other body-mechanics principles that are essential if you are to go through life back-pain-free. Carrying a load of any kind a forearm's length away from you puts ten times as much pressure on the low back as carrying the same load next to you. Try this right now. Pick up this book or another one that is handy and hold it out in front, away from your body. Count very slowly to 60. Does it feel heavier than when you first picked it up? Now bring the book close to your body. Can you feel the difference?

How heavy is a bag of groceries? A sack with just a few items can be heavier than you think, especially if you incorrectly lift that bag out of the trunk. A 20-pound load, lifted from the floor with knees locked, puts 200 lbs. of pressure on the low back. An additional 200 lbs. of pressure is added if the load is held too far away from your body. (Figure 29)

"Close" is the critical ingredient when lifting, pushing, pulling or reaching. (Figure 30) As the load gets farther from you, pressure increases. The ratio is ten times the load when lifting out in front of you; it is fifteen times the load when reaching overhead. (Figure 31) The individual who has a job that

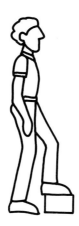

Figure 28
Placing a foot on a stool or ledge gives your back a rest. This position is called the "bar-resting position."

requires manual material handling can very quickly become a spine abuser if he or she does not use good body-mechanics techniques consistently. The term "job" does not necessarily mean your place of employment. You handle many loads in "jobs" outside the work establishment. How about cleaning the garage, bathing the baby or manicuring the yard?

Disc pressure accumulates. A bulging disc is usually the result of wear and tear, and this affects everyone as part of the aging process. But a spine abuser

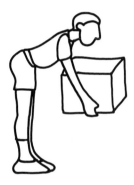

Figure 29
The farther you are from the load, the more pressure you exert on your low back.

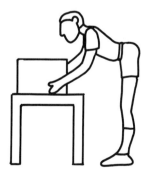

Figure 30
This is a spine abuser in action! Keeping knees locked and lifting a heavy load from far away can trigger back pain.

is a candidate for a serious disc problem, because he or she repeatedly puts excessive pressure on the discs. Knowing the weight of a load is very important, but knowing how to handle the load is even more crucial. In fact, if you do not remember anything else that is written in this book, remember the importance of keeping every load close no matter how light or heavy it is. (Figure 32)

LYING

The study in Sweden covered other common body-mechanics positions that you will want to adopt if you are not using them already. For example, a large part of your 24-hour day is spent sleeping or resting in a prone position.

Have you ever stretched out on the floor while you were having an episode of back pain? (Figure 33) Notice from the illustration that the disc pressure is only 55 lbs. of pressure per square inch, approximately one-half of what it is standing. If you used this body-mechanics position when your back hurt, it probably made you feel semi-comfortable. However, other positions can put even less pressure on the lumbar discs, and they're easy to use.

Do you ever wake up with an aching back? Have you considered buying a new mattress? Before you spend money, consider your sleeping positions.

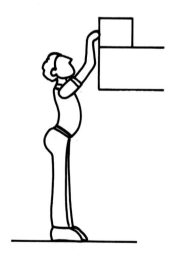

Figure 31
Reaching with locked knees can put 15 times the weight of the load on the lumbar discs.

▼

Almost everyone sleeps on their side sometime during the night, but it is not desirable unless you lie on your side with knees drawn up to your chest (a semi-fetal position). (Figure 34) Then you are putting only 40 lbs. of pressure pressure per square inch on the discs. Lying on your side this way is better than stretching out flat on your back.

However, the body-mechanics position that puts the least amount of pressure on your low back is the "resting" position. (Figure 35) If you are having twinges of back pain or noticeable backache, try this position before you run off to the emergency room. It may solve the problem. The resting position can

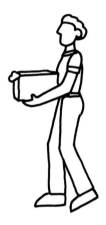

Figure 32
The most important body-mechanics rule to remember: Keep a load close!

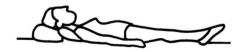

Figure 33
Sleeping on your back or lying flat puts 55 lbs. of pressure per square inch on the low-back discs.

▼

be done anywhere by lying down and placing your feet on pillows, a stool or a piece of furniture. This position can be used for sleeping, or you can use it to take pressure off your lower back while you watch television. Be sure you put a small pillow under your head. If you come home from work with a tired back, try this position for 15 minutes. It is almost guaranteed to make you feel like a new person, or at least a rested one. (Figure 36)

LIFTING

You are probably aware that reams of material have been written on lifting practices, and most of it is very good. If you read any of this information, you already have some basic lifting knowledge, but there may be options you are not aware of. It is important for you to recognize your own capabilities and limitations, and then determine which lifting technique is best for you.

The most commonly known lifting technique is the *squat,* in which you keep your back straight while lifting the load, keeping it close. (Figure 37) There is one problem with this lift. You are off-balance when you begin. Your

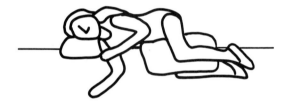

Figure 34
Lying on your side with a pillow between your knees reduces the disc pressure. This position puts only 40 lbs. of pressure on the lumbar discs.

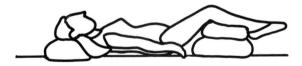

Figure 35
The resting position is the most relaxing for your lower back, because you only put 25 lbs. of pressure on it when you lie this way.

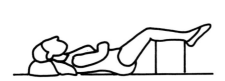

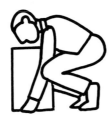

Figure 36
To get comfortable, you can use pillows, a stool or a piece of
furniture under your calves.

Figure 37
Lifting material with your heels off the floor can cause you to
lose your balance.

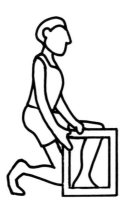

Figure 38
The diagonal stance provides stability and will protect your
back when lifting an object from the floor.

weight is forward, and the load is in front of you. If it should slip, you are likely to fall forward and jerk at the same time.

The *diagonal stance* is a more practical, safer approach. (Figure 38) With one foot in front of the other, you have a wide support base. Keeping one foot flat on the floor also provides additional stability. Anything that is being lifted can be kept close as you stand up, and your foot position allows you to move forward with the object.

If you do not have a great deal of upper-body strength, you can modify this lift further. Keep a knee on the floor for additional leverage as you push off and lift at the same time. (Figure 39)

Other lifting techniques and options will be presented in Chapter 4.

PUSHING AND PULLING

Pushing is easier on your back than pulling in almost every instance. (Figure 40) You can use your arms and legs for leverage when you are pushing more easily than you can when pulling. You can also keep the load close to you and under control.

Sometimes pulling is necessary and pushing is impossible, as when you are handling a water hose, a dog on a leash or kids in a wagon. The problem with pulling is the potential for twisting the low back. (Figure 41) The low back is not designed anatomically to twist, and that can cause serious back pain. Remember how the joints are wider at the bottom of the spine? The narrow

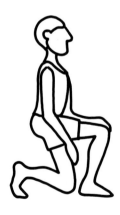

Figure 39
A knee on the floor provides additional leverage when lifting.

joints of the neck allow twisting, but the wide joints in the lumbar spine do not. That's why pulling must be done carefully.

There are several ways to pull without injury. You can pull with both hands to keep your back from twisting. (Figure 42) However, if you are pulling

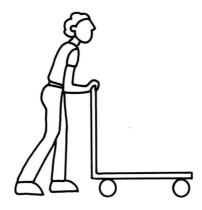

Figure 40
Pushing is usually easier on your back than pulling.

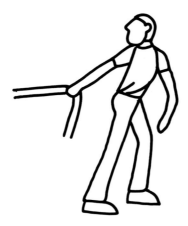

Figure 41
Pulling this way can cause your low back to twist painfully.

something on wheels, you might run over your feet. That could hurt! The safest way to pull is by pulling at your side.

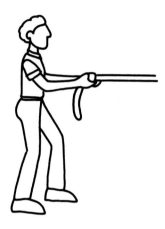

Figure 42
Your legs and arms should provide the leverage when pulling, and the diagonal stance makes pulling easier.

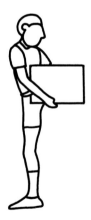

Figure 43
Although your neck and upper back are designed to twist, your low-back discs can be injured by twisting.

PIVOTING

The opposite of twisting is pivoting. Pivoting is the most difficult body-mechanics position to learn, because you have to think about keeping your shoulders, spine and feet going in the same direction. If you add a load to this—especially if it is not moved correctly—you increase the amount of disc pressure on the lumbar spine. Pivoting is essential when you play basketball, dance, shovel or move material on an assembly line. Twisting harms the discs. (Figure 43) Pivoting protects them. Pivoting should be practiced before you start a task. If necessary, look at yourself in a mirror. (Figure 44)

Can you shovel snow without twisting? Keeping your shoulders, hips and feet going in the same direction while moving snow or dirt is tricky. If you are moving the load to the left, start with the diagonal stance, placing your left foot forward. Pick up your left foot, keep the shovel close to you and pivot on the ball of the right foot. If it seems too difficult to manage, start with the diagonal stance and concentrate on moving your shoulders, hips and feet at the same time you are moving the load. Your body should *turn with* the load. (Figures 45, 46) We will present additional pivoting techniques in the next chapter.

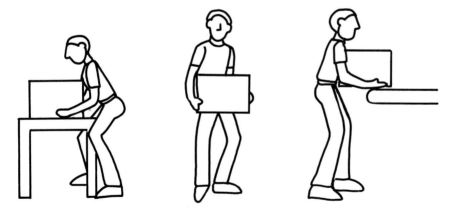

Figure 44
Pivoting is moving your shoulders, hips and feet in the same direction you are moving the load.

WHY DOES JESSE HAVE BACK PAIN?

Can you solve the puzzle? Jesse has back pain, but Bill doesn't. What makes the difference?

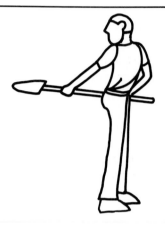

Figure 45
Twisting your low back is asking for injury.

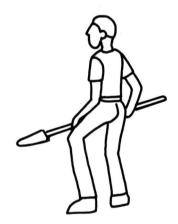

Figure 46
Pivoting is the pain-free alternative to twisting. Move your lead foot with the load, and pivot on the ball of the opposite foot.

For one thing, Jesse sleeps on his stomach or on his side with his legs straight. Bill sleeps on his side with his legs curled up and a pillow between his knees, or he sleeps on his back with a couple of pillows under his legs.

Jesse is 6 feet tall and has to bend over to shave and brush his teeth. Bill is also 6 feet tall, but he opens up a lower-cabinet door and puts a foot in the cabinet while he shaves.

Jesse's car seat is as far back as it can go so he can drive with his legs straight out in front of him. Bill sits down on his seat, pivots his body as he places his legs under the steering wheel, and moves the car seat forward so his knees are higher than his hips.

Jesse keeps his sample products in the trunk of his car. They are in cases with handles, and he must lift them out when he calls on a customer. Jesse usually grabs both of them simultaneously to save time. Bill also keeps his cases in the trunk of his car. However, he keeps a small towel there and puts a knee on the bumper as he picks each case up separately and carefully puts it on the ground.

Both men conduct product demonstrations in clients' offices. Jesse places the cases on the floor and leans over to gather as many samples as he can to show the customer. Bill looks for a place to place the case at waist height and occasionally asks a client if he can use the corner of his desk. Then he doesn't have to lean over. If no space is available, he puts the cases on the floor and bends his knees to pick up the samples.

Jesse stands straight and tall while conversing. This shows he is self-confident. Bill places one foot slightly in front of the other and uses the diagonal stance while tightening his abdominal muscles. He looks self-confident and comfortable at the same time.

Jesse spends three hours in his automobile without a break. Bill watches the time and stops at least once an hour to get out, stretch, and walk around his vehicle.

When the work day is over, Jesse goes home and waters the grass by pulling 200 feet of hose around from the front yard to the back. Bill waters his lawn also. However, he has 50 feet of hose in the front of his house and another 50 feet in the back of his house. He does not have to struggle with pulling hoses all over the place.

Jesse's daughter plays soccer. He slumps over as he watches her for an hour. Bill's son plays football, and Bill takes a stadium seat with him while he observes practice.

After dinner Jesse relaxes by slouching down in his favorite chair to watch television; at 11 p.m. he struggles off to bed. Bill fast-walks at least a mile before dinner and watches television in his recliner with his knees up.

Do you know why Jesse has back pain? Could you suggest changes to improve his daily living activities so he would be more comfortable? How much pressure is he putting on his low back all day?

You are now familiar with basic body-mechanics techniques. Not all of you are built the same way. Not all of you have the same upper-body strength. Some of you are tall and some are short. You are not going to want to lift the same way, nor should you. Posture plays an important role in your everyday activities and your comfort level. Your job and the required activities also influence the kinds of body-mechanics techniques you should be using. You have to determine what body-mechanics positions work the best for you in each situation. We are going to provide you with many options. Then you can pick and choose body-mechanics positions that fit your activities. Not only will you be able to recognize Jesse's problems, but you will be able to recognize your own. ▼

4

▼

Customized Body Mechanics:

Safe Activities for Work, Home and Play

Change of any kind is scary. No one wants to start doing something differently unless the benefits outweigh the aggravation. Fortunately, modifying your body mechanics is much easier than adapting to a new job, a new baby, or a different house. It is also more fun! The only prerequisites are an open mind and the willingness to give it a try. Think of it as "customizing" your movements and activities to your own body and lifestyle. Creativity is helpful, but not necessary for a beginner.

You already know the basic positions that reduce pressure on your back. We will adapt and fine-tune these various body-mechanics techniques to specific activities and chores so you can learn more comfortable ways to do things that are necessary and/or pleasurable.

KITCHEN

Where do you spend most of your active time when you are home? If you are like most of us, you spend it in the kitchen. In most households, the kitchen is the favorite place to congregate. With that in mind, the kitchen will be your first body-mechanics practice area.

Because kitchen activities revolve around eating, let's begin with the moment you get home from the grocery store. *Carrying groceries* into the kitchen and putting them away can be done without hurting your back. Carry one bag at a time unless the bagger has done a terrific job of dispersing the load. (Figure 47) Carry it close to your body. Walk to the counter before you set the bag down—don't try to throw the sack onto the counter. If you do, you

▼

dramatically increase the pressure on your back by shifting the load to an arm's length away—not to mention possibly breaking an item in the bag.

When putting groceries away or preparing meals, you have a couple of good options for *transferring items into or out of the refrigerator*. (Figures 48,

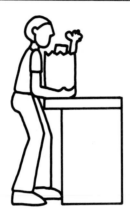

Figure 47
Lifting one sack at a time protects your back.

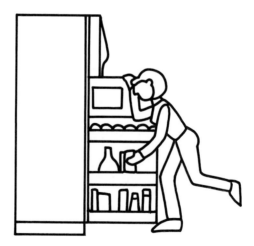

Figure 48
Hold onto the refrigerator door as you reach for food.

49) Because you need to protect your back while reaching, hold onto the door and balance your upper-body weight by extending one leg behind you. This position allows you to reach inside the refrigerator with minimal bending. Or, you can bend your knees a little and place your hand on your thigh for additional support. Your back will feel comfortable if you use either of these positions, and you will be at shelf level.

Once those groceries turn into meals, it is time to think about the body-mechanics position for *sitting and eating.* You have already learned the benefits of sitting with your back supported and your knees higher than your hips, but it doesn't always work when you are trying to put food in your mouth; you are almost required to lean slightly forward. (Figure 50) Pull your seat forward as close to the table as is comfortable. At the same time, drop one knee a little so one foot is behind the other, and scoot forward on your chair. Rest one hand on the table for additional support. (You also can use this technique to prevent low-back discomfort when writing at your desk.)

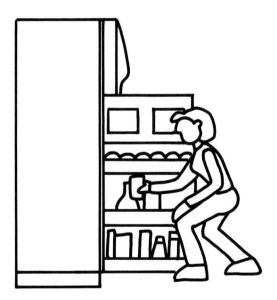

Figure 49
Another method for getting food out of the refrigerator is to place a hand on your thigh to help support your back.

Standing at the kitchen sink, whether to peel potatoes or rinse dishes, is unavoidable. Think about the way you stand. If you stand the wrong way for a long time, you are likely to develop a tired back. Remember the bar-resting position? (Figure 51) To stand comfortably, open a lower-cabinet door and put one foot on the ledge.

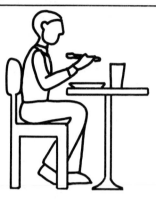

Figure 50
To protect your back when sitting forward, drop one knee so one foot is a little behind the other.

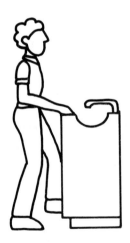

Figure 51
The bar-resting position reduces back pressure when you are preparing meals.

Loading and unloading a dishwasher properly requires a little more thought. Try extending one leg behind you for balance and placing one hand on the counter top for stability. (Figure 52) This position is especially comfortable and easy to use if you are experiencing acute back pain. You can load or unload either from the front or the side, but remember to work straight ahead either way so you don't twist your lower back. Unload the dishes to the counter top, and then put them in the appropriate place.

If not done correctly, *reaching into cupboards* can put a lot of pressure on your back. Pick up pots and pans from low cupboards or drawers by squatting and putting your weight on one or both knees. (Figure 53) The best body-

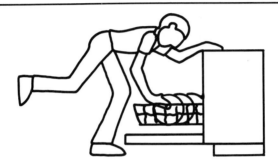

Figure 52
Loading and unloading the dishwasher can be pain-free if you support your back with your hand on the counter top and use your quadriceps muscles.

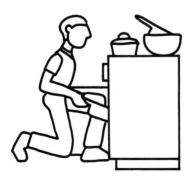

Figure 53
Get down to the level of the cooking equipment.

mechanics technique for this type of task is to get as close to your work level as possible.

Getting up to your work level is as important as getting down to it. A small stool can be a real back-saver. (Figure 54) Consider buying a stool that is movable with wheels and has a spring lock when you stand on it. These are safe and easy to move with your foot. (Moving any item with your foot is a back-saver.)

BATHROOM

Does the position in Figure 55 look familiar? It's the bar-resting position in the bathroom. You can use this position when *shaving or brushing your teeth.* You can also accomplish the same thing by leaning your body and your thighs into the bathroom-sink cabinet. Note the expandable mirror. (Figure 56) Having one of these eliminates the need for leaning over to see yourself.

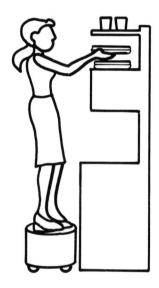

Figure 54
If you have to reach a lot, a small stool can be a good invest-ment.

That mirror is also wonderful for *applying makeup while sitting* at a bathroom vanity or dressing table, but you need to use it differently. If you sit forward on your chair, you put a lot of pressure on the lumbar discs. (Figure

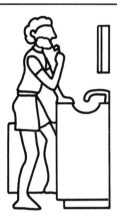

Figure 55
The bar-resting position makes your back feel good while shaving or brushing your teeth.

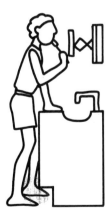

Figure 56
Leaning is an alternative to the bar-resting position. Bend your knees into the cabinet and place your hand on the counter for support.

57) Therefore, move back in your chair so your low back is well-supported. (Figure 58) Getting beautified takes time, so use correct sitting posture. You can't look happy and gorgeous if you have back pain.

Some other bathroom tasks are more difficult. *Bathing the baby or a small child* can be "a real pain" if not done properly. (Figure 59) Place a rug for

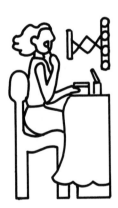

Figure 57
Sitting this way puts a lot of pressure on your low back.

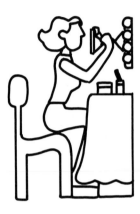

Figure 58
You can be beautiful and comfortable at the same time. An expandable mirror is a back saver.

kneeling next to the tub, and keep the baby as close to the side of the tub as you can. You can support your back in two ways. You can lean against the tub with your thighs and abdomen and/or you can place an arm on the rim of the tub to brace your upper body. Once your child is old enough to understand, make it fun for him or her to stay as close to you as possible. You may get wet, but the benefit to your back will make it worthwhile. When *lifting a small child out of the tub,* face the tub on your knees, or use the diagonal position with one knee

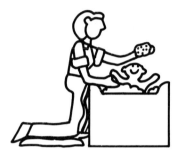

Figure 59
Bathing the baby can be a back killer unless you kneel close to the tub and lean into it.

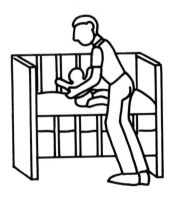

Figure 60
Leaning into the crib is a back saver. Lower the crib side so you don't have to lift the baby over it.

on the floor or the side of the tub. This body-mechanics technique gives you lifting leverage and protects your back at the same time.

BEDROOM

When *lifting a small child out of a crib*, lower the side rail and lean into the bed. (Figure 60) Keep the child as close to you as possible, and lift straight up. Children are often active and squirming, which makes lifting them more difficult. Small children make manual material handling seem easy.

Have your ever tried *making your bed* when you had back pain? If so, you know how painful it can be to lean over from the waist to make the bed.

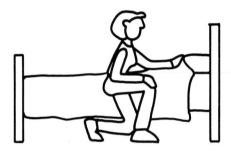

Figure 61
Making the bed without back pain is easy if you get down to a low level.

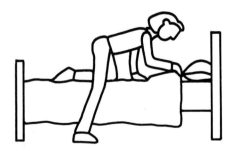

Figure 62
Smooth out the spread after you make the bed this way.

Leaving it unmade can seem like a good idea! Well, you don't have to. You can get down to the level of the bed by kneeling close to the side and making it that way, or you can brace yourself with an arm and a knee on the bed and make it from the top. (Figures 61, 62) The most important factor is to stay close to the bed while making it. Once you have the bedspread on, smooth it out. No one will know the difference. Whatever you do, don't try to make the bed with locked knees. That's back pain on the way to happening.

Getting dressed can occasionally be a problem if your back hurts. When putting on pants or a skirt, try leaning back against the wall. (Figure 63) This body-mechanics position will stabilize you while protecting your low back.

HOUSEKEEPING

Taking out the trash is a never-ending job. Tall garbage cans make for fewer trips, but they are heavy and unwieldy when full. A small wastepaper basket must be emptied much more frequently. No matter which trash container you have, it will be easier to empty if you use your legs for leverage. Bend your knees at the corners of the basket. Reach down, grasp the can by the ridges around the top, and lift straight up. (Figure 64) Empty the trash frequently—especially if in a tall garbage can—so it doesn't get too heavy.

Sweeping is a necessary kitchen and dining area chore—no matter how careful you are, crumbs seem to appear continually. (Figure 65) Sweeping

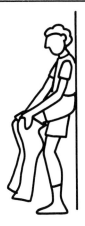

Figure 63
Balancing against the wall protects your back when you are getting dressed.

should be done carefully so you don't twist your lower back. Keep the broom to your side or directly in front of you. Most importantly, keep it close. You can walk with the broom as you sweep.

Vacuuming is a back killer if you're susceptible to back pain. Instead of moving your arm forward and backward, place the handle on your hip or next to your hip and walk with the vacuum cleaner. (Figure 66) This takes a little

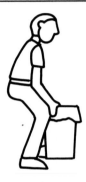

Figure 64
Using your leg muscles for support when lifting the trash basket protects your back.

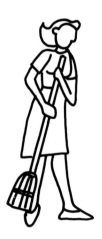

Figure 65
The broom needs to be kept close to your body when you sweep.

practice but becomes easy once you get the hang of it. Don't forget that you can walk backward as well as forward when you are vacuuming. If you have to vacuum under furniture, get down to the level of the area to be cleaned and move the handle slowly. (Figure 67) Keep the handle as close as you can.

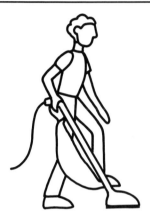

Figure 66
Keeping the vacuum-cleaner handle next to your hip requires practice, but it prevents back pain. Instead of pushing and pulling, walk with it.

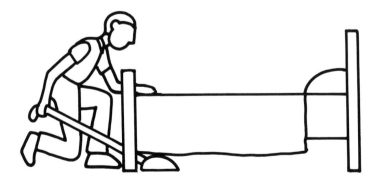

Figure 67
The vacuum-cleaner handle needs to be kept close no matter where you are cleaning.

The body-mechanics position for *dusting or cleaning at low levels* is similar to that of vacuuming at low levels. (Figure 68) You can take pressure off your back by using the diagonal stance and bending your knees a little. This position puts you in a half-squat. Or, you can balance your upper body by putting one leg behind you.

Some jobs such as *scrubbing the floor* aren't fun, no matter how you modify them. (Figure 69) But you can scrub the floor without back pain. Knee pads are a wonderful help. Although they don't protect your back directly, they allow you to kneel comfortably, which takes pressure off the lumbar discs.

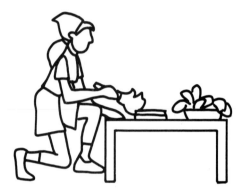

Figure 68
Get close to your work area.

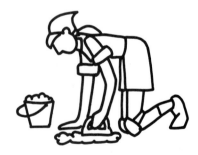

Figure 69
Using knee pads to scrub the floor helps your back *and* your knees.

LAUNDRY

Most washing machines are designed for someone who is very tall, and dryers are designed for someone who is very short. If you are in between, you're going to have difficulty with both pieces of equipment. As you know, wet clothes are heavy. (Figure 70) The obvious solution to *handling wet clothes* is to keep them very, very close. I know you don't want to get wet, but you don't

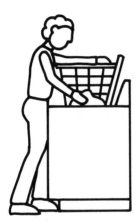

Figure 70
Wet clothes can be very heavy. Lift and carry them close to save your back.

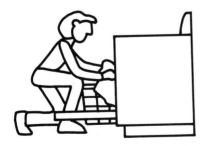

Figure 71
Keep clothes close at the dryer level, too.

want to hurt your back either. Leaning into the washing machine will protect your back.

You will probably have to get down to the level of the dryer door in order to keep your back comfortable. (Figure 71) Small loads are easier to manage than large ones.

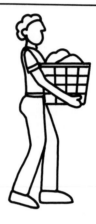

Figure 72
A small load is safer than a large one.

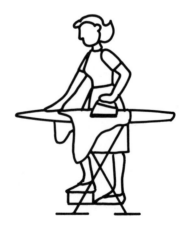

Figure 73
Ironing can be easy if you use the bar-resting position.

When *transporting wet or dry clothes,* use a small basket, and don't try to carry more than is comfortable. (Figure 72) Again, keeping the load close is essential.

Ironing can be comfortable and easy to do if you use a small stool to prop up your foot. (Figure 73) It's the bar-resting position again. If you don't have a stool but you live in a large city, you can make an inexpensive, effective footrest that will last for years by wrapping old telephone books with strapping tape.

SHOP OR GARAGE

The bar-resting position also applies if you are *working in your shop or at a work bench.* (Figure 74) You can stand for a long time when you work if you remember to change feet. A small stool or telephone books are easy to move from one side of the bench to the other. Take advantage of this standing position wherever you are.

If it's not done properly, *working on the car* can cause back pain. (Figure 75) When working under the hood, lean your entire body over the fender to give your upper torso good support. Bend your knees into the side of the car, and place a hand near the grill for added support. If you get tired of this position, try pulling out a small stool and propping up your foot.

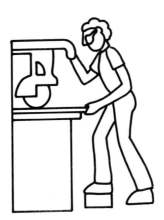

Figure 74
If you have a standing job, look for places to prop your foot.

YARD

There are some outside jobs that require good body-mechanics techniques if you don't want to trigger a backache. Pushing is easier on your back than pulling, but when doing so, you need to use your quadriceps or thigh muscles

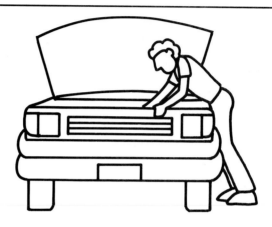

Figure 75
The engine may cause trouble, but your back won't if you remember to lean into the fender.

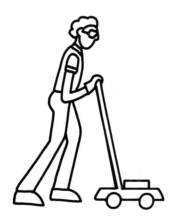

Figure 76
Your arms and legs should provide the leverage when pushing the lawnmower.

instead of your back muscles for leverage. Using the diagonal stance promotes use of your leg muscles and allows you to push or pull without pain.

Mowing the lawn needs to be done carefully. (Figure 76) Think about using your legs—not your back—when pushing the mower, and keep your elbows close to your side. The concept is similar to the body-mechanics position used for vacuuming. Don't let the mower handle get too far away.

The same body-mechanics position applies when *cleaning up with a push broom.* (Figure 77) Keep the push broom next to you, and walk with it like you would with the vacuum cleaner.

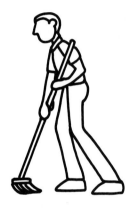

Figure 77
Walk with the broom when cleaning up.

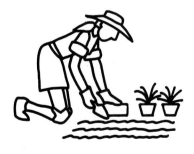

Figure 78
Kneeling protects your back while gardening.

Knee pads will make *planting a garden* or *pulling up weeds* much more comfortable. (Figure 78) To protect your neck and to avoid twisting your lower back, keep your work area directly in front of you.

Edging is one of the most difficult jobs you have to do because it frequently seems to initiate back pain. (Figure 79) Because the electrical edger is held off the ground, it may be more difficult to use than the manual one. No matter which you have, keep the handle as close to your side as possible, and support

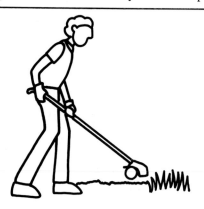

Figure 79
Keep the handle close when edging.

Figure 80
Raking leaves can be fun—if you remember to pivot instead of twist.

it in the middle with your opposite hand to give it direction. The diagonal stance will be beneficial while performing this difficult task.

The smell of burning leaves is one of the pleasant associations we have with autumn. That is, it is pleasant if the job of raking leaves does not initiate back pain. *Raking* needs to be done very carefully to avoid twisting the back. (Figure 80) When raking, keep the leaves and the rake in front of you as much as possible. It isn't always easy, but the benefits to your back outweigh the inconvenience of feeling slightly awkward.

Some yard tasks don't have to be done frequently, but they can mean trouble when they must be done. *Trimming trees* falls into this category. (Figure 81) Instead of leaning into the ladder and arching your back, move your body forward and rest your arm on the top step of the ladder if possible. (Figure 82) The ladder design in the illustrations is excellent for this purpose, because it allows you to support your upper body with your arms.

Remember how hard twisting can be on your lumbar discs? (Figure 83) When *pulling hoses,* place them at your side—as close to your waist or hip as you can—and walk with them. (Figure 84).

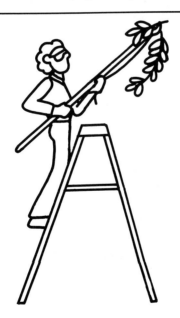

Figure 81
Reaching can trigger back pain, particularly when you use an implement with a handle.

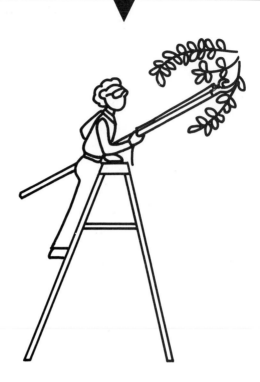

Figure 82
Lean into the ladder for stability, and keep the handle as close
as possible to protect your back.

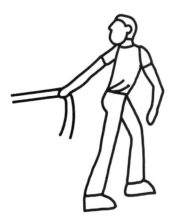

Figure 83
Twisting when pulling hoses can cause a serious back injury.

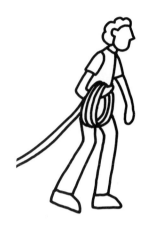

Figure 84
Pull from your side to prevent a twist.

Figure 85
**Pivot when you shovel. Move your body with the load, and
dump the snow to the side.**

Shoveling anything can be tricky, but *shoveling snow* is dangerous for your back if it's not done correctly. Pivoting is not only beneficial, it is essential. (Figure 85) Keep the shovel as close to you as possible, and move the snow to your left or your right. Don't throw the snow in front of you, because the load increases ten times as it moves away from your body. As you shovel to your side, pick up the foot closest to the load and pivot on the opposite foot. (Figure 86) The concept of pivoting is very important to avoid twisting. Basketball players pivot often when trying to keep the ball from being stolen. If they move to the left, they pick up the left foot and turn on the ball of the right foot. When you shovel snow to the left, pick up your left foot, keeping the shovel next to your left thigh. Pivot around on your right foot. Learning to pivot is easier if you concentrate on keeping the load in front of you at all times and as close to you as possible. Also remember to keep your shoulders, hips and feet in a straight line so that your back does not twist. Your entire body should move in unison in the same direction you are moving when shoveling.

Keeping loads close to your center of gravity is always important, and balancing a load also helps protect your back. (Figure 87) Remember this when *carrying firewood*, and use two small totes instead of one if the load is heavy.

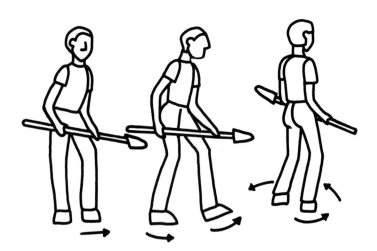

Figure 86
Keep your shoulders in line with your hips and your feet. Your lead foot should move in the same direction as the load.

When *chopping firewood*, use your legs—not your back—for leverage. (Figure 88) The wide diagonal stance will give you good support, and you should keep your arms as close to your body as possible. (Don't forget to wear safety glasses so you don't get wood chips in your eyes.) Some stretching exercises before and after chopping will help you avoid a painful back.

WORKPLACE

Sitting at your desk in the office may be more stressful than sitting at home, but the body-mechanics position is the same. (Figure 89) Sit as close to your desk as possible, and prop your feet on a telephone-book footrest. Hold the telephone by the receiver, because neck pain can occur if you prop the receiver on your shoulder.

The same principles apply when *sitting at a typewriter*. (Figure 90) Place your copy stand in front of you so you will not have to turn your head. This protects your neck as well as your back. Adjust the chair to fit you. Most secretarial chairs are adjustable. Only you know what chair height and tension is comfortable for your back. You may find that you need to vary the height, tension and inclination of your chair fairly often.

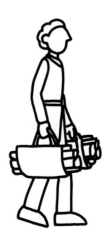

Figure 87
Balance your load by carrying two small items instead of one large one.

When *using a computer terminal,* you must consider the height of the screen. (Figure 91) Telephone books are excellent devices for raising the height of the computer. Adjust the screen to fit your eyes, just like you adjust the chair seat to fit your back. You may also find it necessary to adjust your eyeglasses prescription, particularly if you wear bifocals.

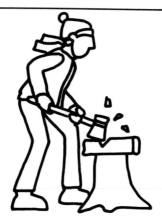

Figure 88
The wide stance gives stability to protect your back from injury.

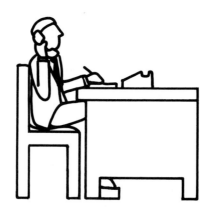

Figure 89
Put your feet on a telephone book or stool to get your knees higher than your hips.

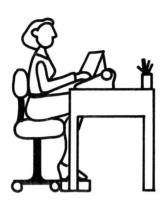

Figure 90
Adjust your chair to fit your back and legs.

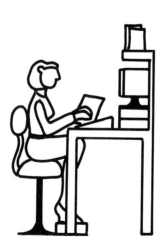

Figure 91
The height of the computer screen will affect your neck and back. The screen should be at eye level.

If your job involves *sitting at an assembly line,* you need good back support. (Figure 92) Many plants have footrests available. If you have one, use it. Your chair may also have rungs where you can place your feet. If you are fortunate enough to have an adjustable chair, use it appropriately. Don't forget to stand whenever possible to vary your body-mechanics position.

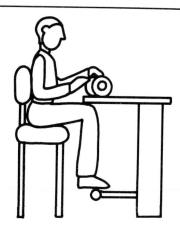

Figure 92
A footrest is beneficial if you have a job that requires sitting for hours.

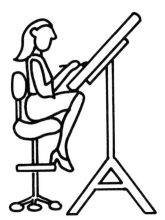

Figure 93
Use the rungs on your chair as a footrest to reduce back pressure.

Sitting at a drafting table gives you a different perspective. (Figure 93) Move the seat as high as you can, and keep the table as close to you as possible.

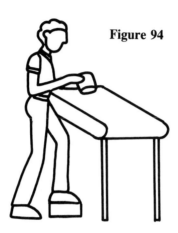

Figure 94

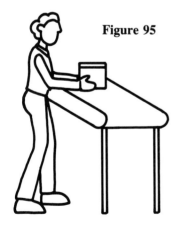

Figure 95

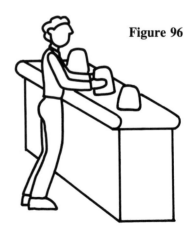

Figure 96

Changing your stance occasionally will decrease disc pressure, and you will be less tired at the end of the day.

Poor sitting posture is not the only body-mechanics position that contributes to back pain. *Standing for long periods* is not likely to cause injury, but it can cause backache and fatigue. If you have a standing job, you have several options. You can use the diagonal or pyramid stance to eliminate low-back pressure. (Figure 94) You can use the bar-resting position (Figure 95), or you can lean into the work counter if it is safe. (Figure 96) All these standing positions reduce the strain on your low back so you are more comfortable at the end of your work day.

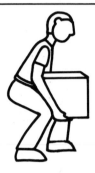

Figure 97
Keeping the load close is mandatory for safe lifting.

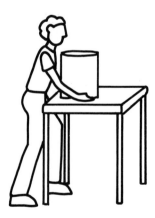

Figure 98
Remember to keep the load close all the way to the drop-off point.

Body-mechanics considerations are essential if your job involves *manual material handling*. These jobs are more likely to cause back injury than most. Manual material handling primarily involves lifting but also includes pushing, pulling, and reaching. When *lifting a load from the floor to a table,* try to keep one foot flat on the floor to balance yourself while you lift the material close to your body. (Figure 97)

When *moving material at waist height,* remember to walk all the way to the deposit point with the load. (Figure 98) Be aware of your options. Some material can be carried safely on your shoulder. (Figure 99) Carrying a load this way keeps it close to your center of gravity and reduces the amount of pressure on your spine.

Reaching can put undue pressure on the low back. (Figure 102) It may sound repetitious. but the wide stance gives you the best protection when *moving material down from a high level.* If the load is difficult to reach, use a stool to get to the level of the load. (Figure 103) Don't carry more than you're capable of moving by yourself. Some jobs may require help from a second person, and you are the expert in determining how much weight you can manage alone.

Remember, you always have options. *Lifting something with a handle,* such as a tool box or pail, can be done correctly by squatting slightly to

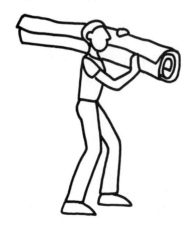

Figure 99
Carry loads as close as possible to your center of gravity. The shoulder-carry is safe for long, narrow material.

balance your body with the weight you are lifting. (Figure 100) Putting your hand on your thigh while lifting will give your back additional support.

"Close" is the key concept in lifting, no matter what the situation, but it is especially true when *climbing stairs and carrying a load.* (Figure 101)

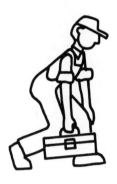

Figure 100
A hand on your thigh will give your back support when lifting an object that has a handle.

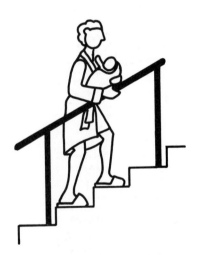

Figure 101
Use three-point contact when climbing: keep two hands and a foot—or two feet and a hand—in contact with surfaces at all times.

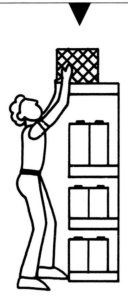

Figure 102
Use the diagonal stance when reaching for a load, and stay close
to the shelving.

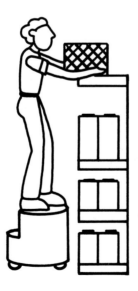

Figure 103
Keep a stool available if reaching is necessary.

Three-point contact is important when climbing. This means that two hands and one foot, or two feet and one hand, are always in contact with the surfaces of stairs and railings. This position helps you avoid a slip or fall.

Pushing is always easier on your back than pulling. (Figure 104) No matter what you're pushing, keep your arms as close to the load as possible, and push

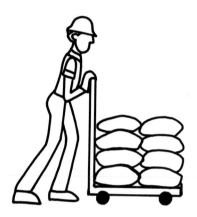

Figure 104
Keep the cart handle close when pushing.

Figure 105
Pushing a stroller or carriage will give you good exercise as long as you use your legs for leverage.

with your legs instead of your back. This body-mechanics principle is the same one you use when mowing the lawn. Although a baby in a stroller may be lighter, good body mechanics are still necessary. (Figure 105)

Remember that *pulling* can cause twisting if you don't do it carefully. Keep the handle next to your side, and balance your load if you are carrying two items. (Figure 106) Another pulling option is to put both hands behind you to avoid a twist. However, remember to protect your heels. (Figure 107)

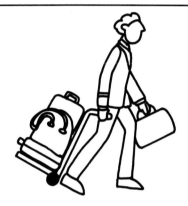

Figure 106
Pull the load at your side to avoid twisting your lumbar spine.

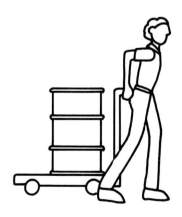

Figure 107
Placing both hands on the handle is a safe way to pull, but do not run over your heels with the cart.

TRAVEL

Have you had back pain after *driving or riding in the car* for long periods? Unfortunately, many car seats are not designed to be especially comfortable. Start thinking about how you sit and also how you might modify the seat position. If your car seat is uncomfortable, use a commercial back support or roll up a hand towel or bath towel and put it behind your lower back as a back support. (Figure 108) Remember to move the car seat forward close enough so your knees are higher than your hips. Most people sit with their car seats too far back, and they have to reach for the steering wheel. Moving your car seat forward even one notch may help.

When *getting into and out of the car,* pivot your entire body around before you stand up. (Figure 109) Once you have turned around, put one hand on the steering wheel and the other on the door frame to give you additional support as you stand up.

Lifting children out of the back seat can be difficult. Although there is no easy way to do this, the diagonal stance helps. (Figure 110) This position allows you to get as close to the child as you physically can and lift him or her up before you back out of the car. Once they can walk, let them help as much as possible.

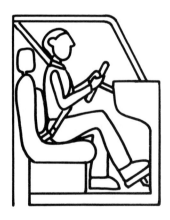

Figure 108
A back support can be helpful when driving, but you need to try it out and make sure it fits your back.

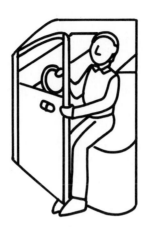

Figure 109
To avoid twisting your low back, pivot your body when getting
into and out of your vehicle.

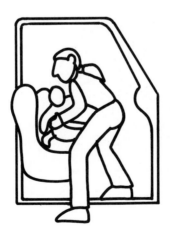

Figure 110
Use the diagonal stance when lifting children out of the car.

▼

Lifting objects out of the trunk may be difficult, but it's not nearly as hard as getting children out of the back seat of the car. (Figure 111) Give yourself a mechanical advantage by placing your knee on the bumper. (To protect your clothing, keep a small towel in the trunk of the car to place on the bumper.) This position is also beneficial if you have to work under the hood from the front of the car. Take one bag or suitcase out at a time. Don't try to pick up more than you can carry comfortably.

Carrying suitcases is easier on your back when you pack two small ones rather than one large one. (Figure 112) Frequently, airports offer very little baggage assistance. If you have to check one suitcase, you might as well check two.

Have you ever looked at an airplane seat from the side? If not, do so and you will immediately understand why it is so uncomfortable. It is designed with an unnatural curve that seems to compound the back-pain problem. (Figure 113) If you are a frequent airplane traveler, there are several things you can do to make *sitting in an airplane seat* more comfortable. Use one or two small pillows behind your back. If that is uncomfortable, ask the flight attendant for a blanket, and fold it to make a back rest. The other thing you can do is take a briefcase or overnight case with you, and place it under the seat in front of you until you are airborne. Then place it under your feet to get your knees higher

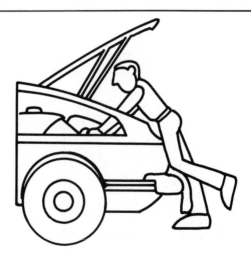

Figure 111
When lifting loads out of the back of the car, lean into the trunk or place a knee on the bumper.

▼

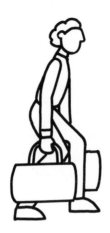

Figure 112
Carrying two small suitcases is better for your back than a large one.

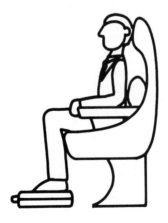

Figure 113
A pillow or two may help your back in the plane seat. Your briefcase can become a footrest once you are airborne.

than your hips. Modifying your body-mechanics position like this takes a great deal of pressure off your lumbar discs, and your back will be pain-free when you arrive at your destination.

LEISURE ACTIVITY

After all your work and travel, a little stretching will feel good. You can combine that with rest time.

When *sitting in front of the television,* get your knees higher than your hips. (Figure 114) An ottoman is helpful for this purpose. If you have a recliner, lean back and put your feet on the footrest with your knees bent.

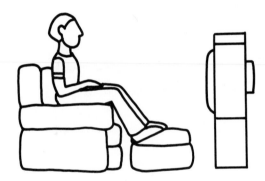

Figure 114
Watching television does not require slouching. Give your back good support, and get your knees higher than your hips.

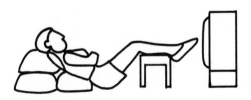

Figure 115
Comfort and entertainment is possible at the same time if you use this resting position.

If your back is really tired, lie down on the floor and put your feet up on an ottoman or stool. (Figure 115) Your head may need to be a little higher so you can see the television, so arrange a couple of pillows under your head and shoulders for comfort.

If you prefer *reading* to watching television, situate yourself on the sofa with plenty of pillows for back and neck support. (Figure 116) Getting your knees up will add to your comfort level. Try putting a couple of pillows under your knees to support them.

For *reading or watching television* in bed, you also need to think about your body-mechanics positions. (Figure 117) Use the same kind of positioning that

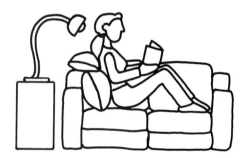

Figure 116
Reading like this is comfortable for your back and neck.

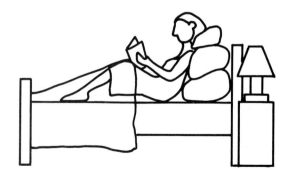

Figure 117
Position the pillows carefully to support your neck and back.

you did when sitting on the couch and reading. Arrange the pillows so you have good back support as well as neck support. You can also put a pillow or two under your knees to reduce the disc pressure.

SLEEPING

Good sleeping positions make a big difference in how you feel when you get out of bed in the morning. Although nothing is carved in stone decreeing that only one position is the best, it is hard to improve on sleeping on your back with a pillow or two under your knees. (Figure 118) If you have osteoporosis, you may want to put an additional pillow under your shoulder blades when lying on your back. However, not all of us can sleep on our backs, and you may find that position impossible or uncomfortable. If so, try sleeping on your side with a pillow between your knees. (Figure 119) If that is uncomfortable, roll up a small hand towel and put it under your waist while lying on your side. The towel will also add support. Most people find this position very comfortable. You can also change positions during the night.

If you are a dedicated stomach sleeper, try putting a pillow under your abdomen. (Figure 120) This takes some getting used to but is well worth the effort to avoid waking up every morning with a sore back. You may want to use a smaller pillow for your head than you have been using in the past simply because it will be more comfortable.

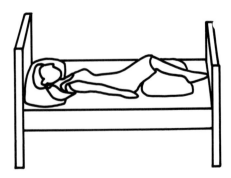

Figure 118
Pillows under your knees reduce back pressure and let you sleep comfortably.

COUGHING AND/OR SNEEZING

This situation can occur quickly and unexpectedly anywhere, and coughing or sneezing often initiates an episode of back pain. If you feel a cough or sneeze starting, brace yourself against a wall or a piece of furniture. (Figure 121) If you are in an open space, use the diagonal stance and support your upper body with an arm across your abdomen. (Figure 122)

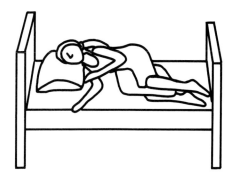

Figure 119
Lying on your side with a pillow between your knees contributes to a restful night.

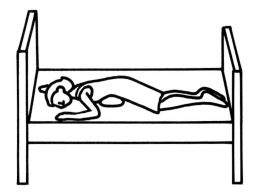

Figure 120
A small pillow under your abdomen may allow you to sleep on your stomach without back pain.

NECK POSITIONS

Although the focus of this book is the care of the lumbar spine, it is virtually impossible to take care of your low back without also using good body-mechanics and posture techniques to protect your neck and upper back.

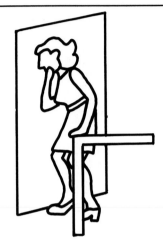

Figure 121
When coughing or sneezing, brace yourself against a wall or a piece of furniture.

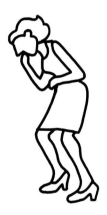

Figure 122
Flexed knees and an arm across your body will support you when you cough or sneeze.

If you have experienced episodes of neck pain, you need to think about the position of your head in relation to your shoulders. You may have inadvertently developed a *head-thrusting* posture. Head-thrusters are prone to stand with a sagging abdomen and drooping shoulders. (Figure 123) Instead, concentrate on standing straight with your ears directly over your shoulders,

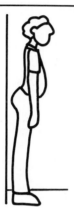

Figure 123
Head-thrusters have neck pain due to poor posture.

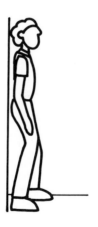

Figure 124
Stand and move as if you are lined up at the wall. Good posture protects your entire spine.

chin tucked in, and abdominal muscles tight. (Figure 124) This posture technique must be practiced consciously to become a habit.

You may also be thrusting your head when you are sitting at your desk, reading, driving or watching television. If so, neck pain is likely. (Figures 125, 126, 127) You will be more comfortable if you use pillows behind your back or a commercial back support and tuck your chin in toward your chest. This is referred to as the *turtle position* because you actually tuck your chin and bring your head back in line with your neck and shoulders. (Figures 128, 129, 130)

Figure 125

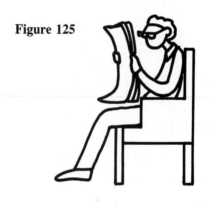

Figure 127

Figure 126

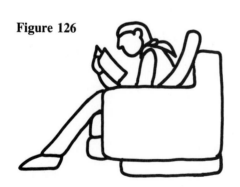

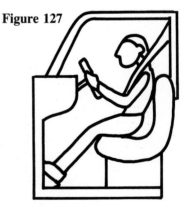

Bad habits can develop quickly, leading to pain in the neck and upper back.

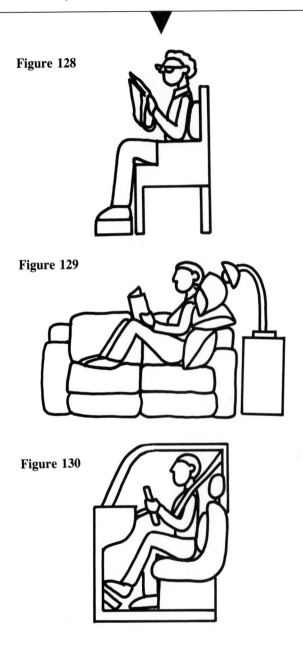

Figure 128

Figure 129

Figure 130

The "turtle" position will keep you comfortable. Pull your chin in toward your chest so your head is directly over your shoulders.

Do not work with your head bent forward against gravity. Remember to change positions every 20 minutes to reduce the chances of neck strain or pain.

Avoid reading an unfolded newspaper, especially if you wear bifocals. Instead keep the newspaper folded and directly at eye level. Another tip for avoiding neck pain is to avoid sitting near the front of the theater or auditorium. This position causes you to tilt your head backward and can trigger an episode of neck pain.

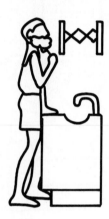

Figure 131
Good body mechanics protect your entire spine.

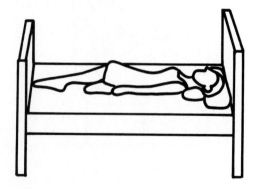

Figure 132
A towel roll under your neck supports your cervical spine.

The use of an expandable mirror allows you to keep your body straight and your chin tucked while shaving. (Figure 131) Again, practice is important.

If you wake up with neck pain, try altering your pillow situation. If you sleep on your back, use a very thin pillow and make sure your head is well-aligned. A rolled-up hand towel under your neck also may give you extra support and make you more comfortable. (Figure 132) If you sleep on your

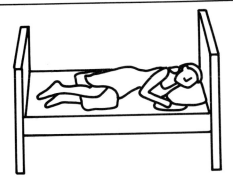

Figure 133
Place your pillow so it supports your head, neck and shoulders.

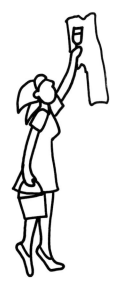

Figure 134
Neck pain is likely if you paint the walls this way.

side, a thicker pillow may be comfortable. (Figure 133) Your head should be in line with your shoulders.

You know that back pain is possible when reaching overhead, but so is neck pain. You are particularly vulnerable if you are in a position where your neck

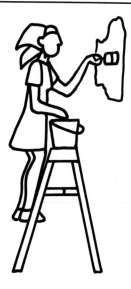

Figure 135
Work at eye level to reduce pressure on your neck.

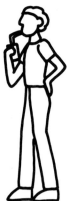

Figure 136
Using a straw for drinking out of cans and bottles prevents neck extension.

is bending backward. (Figure 134) Working at eye level will eliminate the problem. (Figure 135)

The use of a straw when drinking out of bottle or can—and proper use of the telephone receiver—is also going to keep your neck in an appropriate position to protect you. (Figures 136, 137)

. . . AND FOR EVERYTHING ELSE YOU DO

Although we may have missed some things that you do on a day-to-day basis, you should be able to see yourself in many of the situations we've covered. For activities that we haven't covered, you can figure out safe movements that protect your back if you know basic body-mechanics principles:

1. Sit with your knees higher than your hips.

2. Practice standing with one foot slightly in front of the other, knees bent just a little, abdominal muscles tight and buttocks tucked. This is the diagonal or pyramid stance that takes pressure off your low back.

3. Keep everything close. That means you get close to your work level, no matter where you are, up high or down low. Work straight ahead to keep everything close.

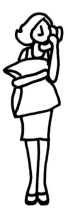

Figure 137
Keep the telephone receiver off your shoulder; hold the phone up to your ear.

▼

4.   Push whenever possible. Use your legs for leverage.

5.   If you must pull an object, keep it at your side or directly behind you. Don't twist.

6.   Lift with your thigh and abdominal muscles instead of your back.

7.   Carry reasonable loads. Get help if the load seems difficult or unmanageable.

Changing everyday habits is not easy. It takes a concentrated effort and a lot of practice as well as commitment to taking care of your back. Because you are the back owner, you are the only one who can decide if the modification is worth it. It will take several months of conscious practice for the use of good body mechanics to become automatic. Transferring techniques from one situation to another also takes some effort. The reward is control of your pain.

▼

▼

5

Do I Have To?

Exercises for the Back-Pain Sufferer

"She is crazy! My back is killing me and she expects me to do exercises! I can't sit for more than a few minutes at a time, I can't sleep, I can't even stand very well, and she wants me to try something called a "pelvic tilt"? Dr. Johnson told me to come to Back School, but he certainly didn't tell me I was expected to exercise in my present condition.

"Well, here goes—knees bent, hand underneath my back at my waist, press the small of my back into my hand, slightly tilt my pelvis and feel my abdominal muscles tighten. Actually that feels pretty good. I don't know if the pelvic tilt is a real exercise, but it is easy and comfortable. Sure, I can do five of those. A knee-to-chest stretch? One knee at a time? If it doesn't hurt any more than the pelvic tilt, I'll try that too. Besides, I would feel silly if the other people in the class could do this and I was the only one who wouldn't try. This isn't bad at all. In fact, I hate to admit it, but maybe my back feels a little better already."

Exercise. The word alone can make you cringe. It conjures up many mental images: slim young women in leotards, young men who look like Greek gods, Jane Fonda, the New York marathon. Which category do you relate to? If you are like most people, the answer is, "None." However, exercise that protects your back by maintaining flexibility and strength does not have to be strenuous. You don't have to be young—you don't even have to be thin. It is an equal opportunity situation.

Exercise for the back-pain victim is a relatively new treatment that has proved very successful. Only a few years ago, doctors advised total bed rest for every patient with back pain. Although most recovered in a few weeks, they were deconditioned and often less able than before to perform their jobs at work or at home. Because back pain is such a frightening experience, it is understandable that a person in pain does not want to move. But we know that suitable exercise can be tremendously beneficial.

To help you progress sensibly with an appropriate exercise regimen, we will describe common back-pain symptoms and the safest exercises for each condition. The floor exercises are designed primarily for stretching and strengthening muscles. They will make you more flexible, which is of proven benefit in protecting you against recurring problems. Muscles that are properly stretched work more effectively. Appropriate exercises also decrease the muscle spasm that usually accompanies back pain.

Before we introduce you to specific exercises, there is one caution. If you start an exercise program after a period of inactivity, you may become sore. Some discomfort is to be expected if you are suddenly using body parts that are "rusty" from disuse. However, if any of the following exercises causes pain, discontinue it immediately. You are the back owner, so it is up to you to listen to your back. Any exercise program should be started slowly and continued at a reasonable pace. You will not gain anything by trying to do it all at once as a weekend athlete.

We recommend that you begin the floor exercises with five repetitions of each until you feel confident that your back can tolerate more than that. In the beginning it is better to practice five repetitions two or three times a day than 10 or 15 repetitions all at one time.

BACK PAIN WITHOUT LEG PAIN

The following exercises are for you if you are experiencing *back pain without leg pain*. These should be done slowly and deliberately, five repetitions at a time, twice a day.

Pelvic Tilt (Figures 138, 139)

Lie on your back with knees bent so your feet are flat on the floor. Place your hand under your low back and slowly press against your hand with the small of your back. You should feel your stomach muscles tighten as you flatten your back against the floor. Once you feel this sensation, you can remove your hand. Think about pressing your weight into the floor. Slowly count to five and relax for a moment before you repeat the exercise.

Modified Sit-up (Figures 140, 141, 142)

Begin with the pelvic tilt. Place your hands by your side. Lift your head so your chin almost touches your chest. Lift your shoulders off the floor as you

Figure 138

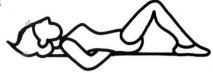

Figure 139

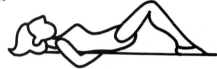

Pelvic Tilt

Figure 140

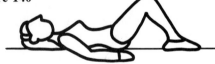

Figure 141

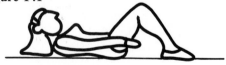

Figure 142

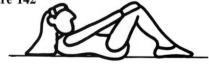

Modified Sit-up

reach for your knees. Touch the top of your knees with your fingers, and hold for the count of two. Then lower your shoulders slowly to the floor. Keep your chin tucked. Lower your head slowly to the floor. Be sure not to arch your back during any part of this exercise, and do not raise your back, only your shoulders. This exercise helps strengthen your abdominal muscles so they give better support to the front of your spine. Once you are comfortable with this exercise, try holding the sit-up position for the count of five.

Double Knee-to-Chest (Figures 143, 144)
This exercise can also be identified as the *low-back stretch*. Begin with the pelvic tilt. Slowly bring one knee toward your chest. Hug your knee tightly enough to feel a mild stretch in your low back. Hold for the count of 30. Lower your leg and repeat with the other leg. Once you are comfortable with one knee at a time, try bringing both knees to your chest—but bring one knee up first and then the other. Do not arch your back during any part of this exercise. The double knee-to-chest exercise is designed to stretch low back muscles to their normal lengths. Lower one leg at a time.

Hamstring Stretches (Figures 145, 146, 147, 148, 149)
The old saying "variety is the spice of life" applies to the hamstring stretch. There are many ways to accomplish the same results, so the choice is yours. Begin with the stretch that is easiest for you and progress to the most difficult.

The hamstring muscle runs from the hip down the back of your thigh to your knee. This exercise is designed to give your back and hip additional flexibility. This exercise can be done lying, standing or sitting, so start with the *lying*

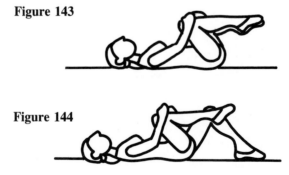

Figure 143

Figure 144

Double Knee-to-Chest

Figure 145

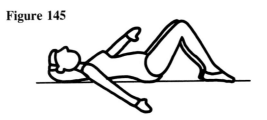

Figure 146

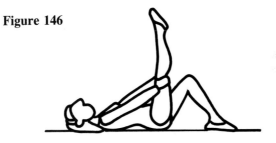

Lying Hamstring Stretch

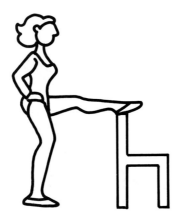

Figure 147
Standing Hamstring Stretch

hamstring stretch. (Figures 145, 146) Lie on your back with knees bent so your feet are flat on the floor. Raise your leg slowly as shown by clasping your hands around the back of the knee to support the lower thigh. Slowly straighten the knee, and feel a stretch in the back of your leg. Hold for the count of three and relax. Repeat with the opposite leg.

The *standing hamstring stretch* can be done easily with a table or a chair back. (Figure 147) Stand with one leg propped on a table or the back of a chair. chair. Bend the leg you are standing on until you feel a mild stretch under the thigh of the leg on the chair. Hold for a count of three. This may be a more difficult exercise, but will give you some variety if you are tired of being on the floor.

The third option, the *sitting hamstring stretch,* is to sit on the floor with one leg bent and the other almost straight. (Figures 148, 149) Lean forward slowly over the bent leg until you feel a mild stretch under the other thigh. Hold for a count of three. Repeat with the other leg. You do not want to feel severe pain—only a mild stretch—with this exercise.

Figure 148

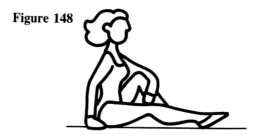

Figure 149

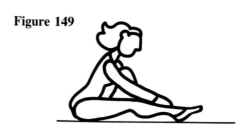

Sitting Hamstring Stretch

PAIN DOWN YOUR LEG

The next set of exercises are for you if you are experiencing *pain down your leg*. Also, if you are a candidate for osteoporosis or have been diagnosed with the disease, these are appropriate. They are extension (backward bending) exercises rather than flexion (forward bending) exercises. Furthermore, they will promote good posture.

Press-up (Figures 150, 151)

Lie on your stomach. Place your hands on the floor at shoulder level. Push up with your arms, *leaving your hips on the floor!* Go up as far as you can, and return to the floor. Do not stay in this position. If you have leg pain, try this exercise 10 to 12 times every two to three hours for the first 24 hours. At that time you will know if the exercise is helping. If your pain should become worse, *discontinue*. If your pain decreases, do 10 to 12 press-ups three times a day. This is also a good exercise for you if you have poor posture or have been sitting or leaning forward for a long time.

Hump and Sag (Figures 152, 153)

This is a good exercise for stretching and strengthening. Start this exercise on your hands and knees. Slowly make a mountain out of your back, similar to an angry cat; then let it slowly sag like an old horse. Repeat this exercise five to 10 times. Once you are comfortable with this exercise, you can progress to the donkey kick.

Figure 150

Figure 151

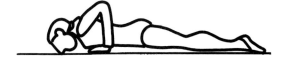

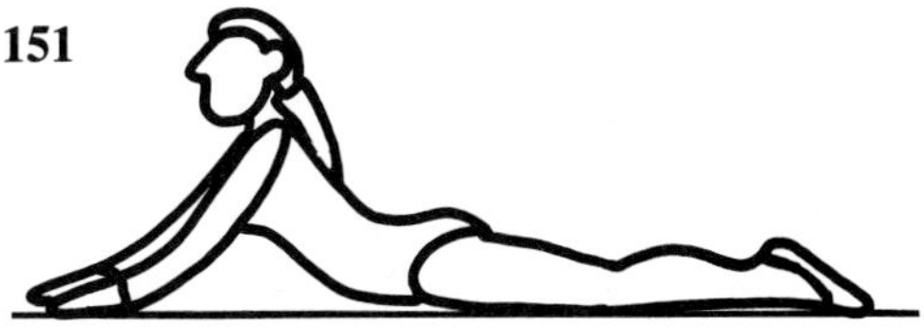

Press-up

Donkey Kick (Figures 154, 155, 156)

If you are comfortable doing the hump and sag, try this exercise. Start on your hands and knees. Keep your head down, bringing one knee to your elbow. Then very slowly push the leg out behind you. Watch underneath your body and do not lose sight of your toes. You don't want to arch your back, and you need to keep your legs in line with your hip. Repeat with the other leg. If you are feeling especially athletic, you can balance your body by reaching with an opposite leg and arm while doing this exercise. However, you must not arch your back. If this exercise causes pain, do not continue.

EXERCISES AFTER PAIN SUBSIDES

Once you have recovered from your episode of back pain, it will be very beneficial if you continue with some kind of stretching and strengthening program. It is always easy to find excuses not to exercise, but 10 or 15 minutes of these types of exercises can make a big difference in the way you and your back feel.

Because flexibility is critical to your general conditioning, structure your program with a combination of flexion and extension exercises. Four sets of exercises will be adequate, but they must be done at least four times a week to be effective. In the beginning, choose from the preceding group; add others

Figure 152

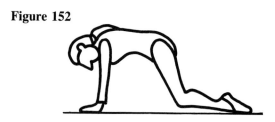

Figure 153

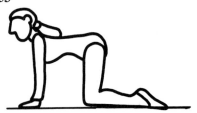

Hump and Sag

Figure 154

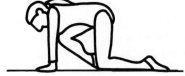

Figure 155

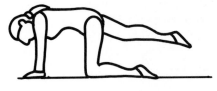

Figure 156

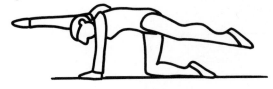

Donkey Kick

from the following list as you wish. The next group of exercises will be beneficial because they will strengthen your legs and abdominal muscles, which will in turn provide support for your spine.

Ten repetitions of four or five different exercises will give you variety so you won't get bored, and keep you flexible and strong. This routine will not take more than 20 minutes. Of course, 30 minutes of exercise five times a week would be even better.

The following are leg-strengthening exercises. Strong legs help protect your back. They make it easier for you to perform many of the proper body-mechanics techniques.

Straight-leg Raise (Figures 157, 158)
Lie on your back with one knee bent so your foot is flat on the floor and the other leg is straight. Perform the pelvic tilt, and hold it as you raise the straight leg only eight inches off the floor. Hold for five seconds, then slowly lower your leg and relax the pelvic tilt. Be sure you keep your foot flat rather than pointing your toe. Not only will this strengthen your legs, it will also strengthen your abdominal muscles.

Leg Lift (Figures 159, 160, 161)
Leg lifts also offer some variety. Lie on your side with your bottom leg bent slightly under you. Place your top arm in front of you on the floor for support.

Figure 157

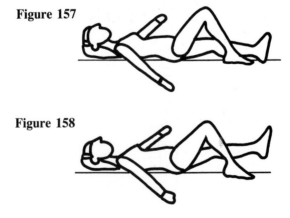

Figure 158

Straight-leg Raise

▼

Align your shoulders and hips. Slowly raise your upper leg until it is above shoulder height and lower slowly. Repeat five times. Turn over and repeat this exercise on the other side with the opposite leg. Make sure your shoulders stay in line with your hips.

Figure 159

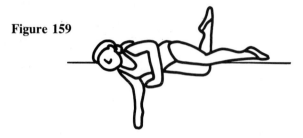

Figure 160

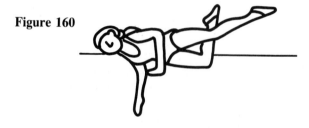

Figure 161

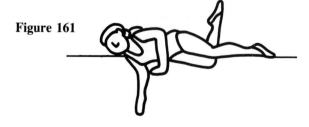

Leg Lift

▼

Wall Slide (Figures 162, 163)

Place your back flat against a wall, and bend your knees as though you are in a sitting position. Start with knees only slightly bent and try to hold the position for two minutes. When this becomes easy after several sessions, begin bending your knees more to work toward holding it in a sitting position. This exercise is guaranteed to make your thighs sore at first, but it is worth the

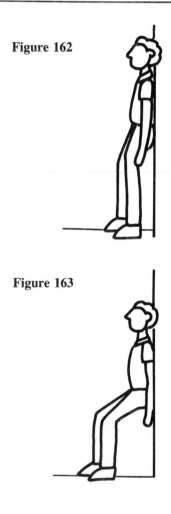

Figure 162

Figure 163

Wall Slide

aggravation. If you ski, this exercise is particularly helpful because it strengthens your all-important quadriceps (thigh) muscles.

Partial Squat (Figures 164, 165)
This is probably the easiest exercise of all, but don't be deceived, it is very helpful for your legs. Take time throughout the day to just bend your knees slightly in the diagonal stance and hold that position for 15 to 30 seconds. If you are trying this at work, you might warn your peers that you are doing some leg-strengthening exercises. Some of them may join you.

Figure 164

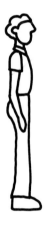

Figure 165

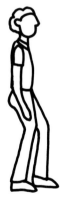

Partial Squat

STRETCHING

Although specific exercises have been recommended for your back and legs, stretching before any activity increases your mobility and flexibility. The next two are excellent for improving posture. They should be done often if you must sit a great deal or have tense back and shoulder muscles. In fact, these will probably feel so good that you will want to do them several times a day.

Extension Stretch (Figure 166)

Simply stand up from your sitting position, bend your knees slightly, place your hands on the back of your waist and stretch backward while looking at the ceiling. Hold for the count of five and then slowly stand up. This exercise can be done anytime, anyplace and will improve your posture.

Almost Elbow Touch (Figure 167)

Almost-elbow touches are also excellent for posture improvement. Stand up straight and simply try to touch your elbows while they are behind you. Most people cannot touch their elbows, but the stretch is beneficial. Hold the position for the count of five and then relax.

Shoulder Stretch and Hug (Figures 168, 169)

Other good stretches for the neck and upper back are shoulder stretches and hugs. Interlock your fingers, raise your hands over your head and simply

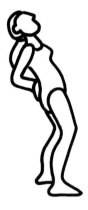

Figure 166
Extension Stretch

stretch upward. When you have completed that stretch, give yourself a hug by wrapping your hands around your shoulders and hugging yourself tightly. This will stretch out those tense, tight upper back or thoracic muscles.

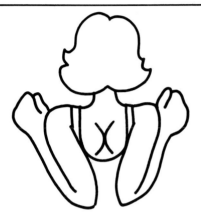

Figure 167
Almost-elbow Touch

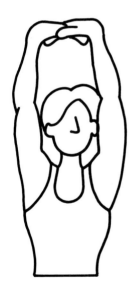

Figure 168
Shoulder Stretch

EXERCISES AS YOU INCREASE YOUR ACTIVITY

The following stretches will help if you're going to increase your activity. Many of these are variations of exercises that have already been presented, but they give you some options and keep your stretching program interesting. Don't try to incorporate all of the stretches in your exercise program. Concentrate on those you like and that support the activities you want to pursue.

Progressive Quadriceps Stretch (Figures 170, 171, 172, 173, 174)
Start in a kneeling position. Place your hands on the floor, and bring one knee toward your elbow. Stretch the other leg out behind you, bend it upward, and stretch it by gently pulling with the opposite hand. Progressive exercises are done slowly and deliberately. Hold the position for the count of five. Repeat with the opposite leg. This exercise is especially appropriate for activities involving fast walking or running.

Calf Stretch (Figures 175, 176, 177)
Calf stretches are excellent for fast walking or running activities—and very important for anyone who wears high heels. Calf muscles and hamstring muscles shorten easily, and these exercises prevent that from happening. They can be done almost anywhere. Lean against a wall with your hands at a comfortable height. Place your feet in a diagonal stance. Bend your forward knee as you place your weight on the back leg and press your foot flat on the floor. You should feel your calf muscle stretch. Hold this position for the

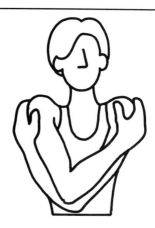

Figure 169
Shoulder Hug

Figure 170

Figure 171

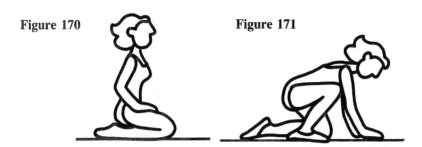

Figure 172

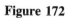

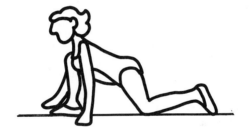

Figure 173

Figure 174

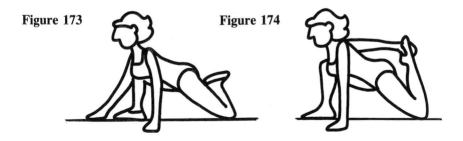

Progression of Quadriceps Stretching

count of five. You may accomplish the same stretch by leaning on a table. Be sure you flatten your back foot. Calf stretches can also be done effectively by placing your foot on a stair and pressing downward. The same calf stretching sensation should occur.

Because high heels tend to make the hamstring muscles and calf muscles shorten, women in particular should do at least one set of these everyday.

Figure 175

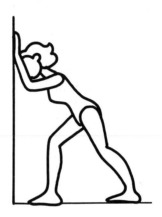

Figure 177

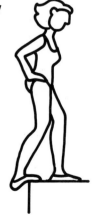

Figure 176

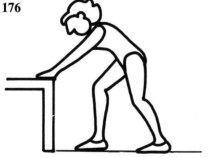

Calf Stretches

However, cowboy boots have high heels also, so women are not the only ones who are susceptible to shortened calf muscles.

Low-back Stretch (Figure 178)
This exercise is similar to the knee-to-chest stretch, and will accomplish the same thing—but in a standing position. Don't try this unless you are confident of your balance. Slowly bring one knee toward your chest, and grasp it with your hands. Hold for a count of three. Change feet. This allows the low-back muscles to stretch. Five repetitions will help relax tired, tense muscles.

Thigh Stretch (Figures 179, 180)
Because total body flexibility protects you, you should also stretch your inner-thigh muscles. Lie on your back. Put the bottoms of your feet together as you move your legs slowly up and then back down toward you. Keep the bottoms of your feet together. As you widen your legs, you will feel the stretch. Do not strain your thigh muscles. Hold your legs in a gentle stretching position for the count of five.

Once you have become flexible, you can try a variation. Sit with your feet together, and press downward gently with your elbows on the insides of your knees. Hold for the count of five, and relax. Do not do the sitting thigh stretches if you are experiencing back pain.

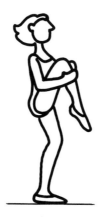

Figure 178
Low-back Stretch

WATER EXERCISES

If you have access to a swimming pool or a spa, take advantage of it. Water is a wonderful muscle relaxer and can help increase your flexibility. Water exercises are easy to do because the force of gravity is less when you are immersed in water. The following exercises will feel good whether you have an episode of back pain or are simply using them to increase your mobility and prevent recurring injury.

Knees to Chest (Figures 181, 182)

Stand chest-deep in water, and hold on to the side of the pool with one hand. Bring your opposite knee up and use that arm to hold it against your chest for the count of ten. Repeat very slowly five times. Switch sides, and repeat the exercise with the opposite leg. This exercise will allow your back muscles to stretch to their normal length. If you are comfortable in the water and can swim, you might want to try the knee-to-chest rotation exercise. Back up to the pool's edge, stretch out both arms, and hold on. Bring both knees up toward your chest, and slowly move your knees from side to side. This is a very controlled exercise that should be done slowly to be effective. This will stretch your back muscles and the muscles at your waist.

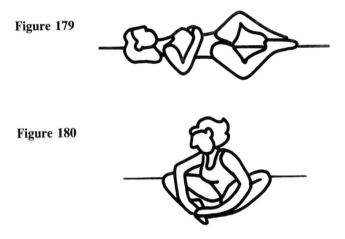

Figure 179

Figure 180

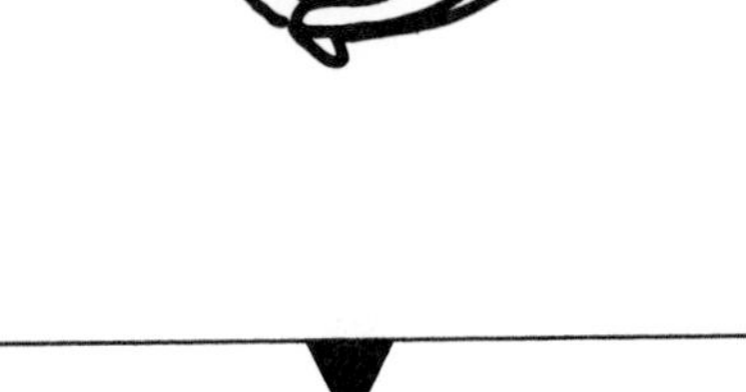

Thigh Stretches

Leg Raise (Figures 183, 184)

Leg raises strengthen your abdominal muscles and stretch your hamstring muscles.

Stand comfortably in the water, holding on to the side of the pool with one hand. *Slowly and deliberately* raise one leg straight in front of you, then lower it slowly. Do five of these and change sides. Once you are comfortable with leg raises, add a knee bend to strengthen your quadriceps muscles. Slowly bend the supporting leg as you raise the other. Hold for the count of five, straighten up slowly, and lower your leg slowly. Start with five repetitions, and work up to ten on each side.

Figure 181

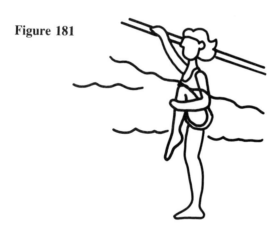

Figure 182

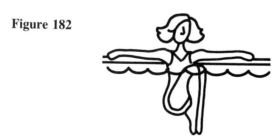

Knees to Chest

Extension Stretch (Figure 185)

Face the side of the pool, holding on with both hands. Slightly bend one leg while slowly kicking the other out behind you. Repeat ten times with each leg.

EXERCISE CLASSES

(Figure 186) Floor exercises tend to be boring, so unless you are a well-disciplined individual, you may find that the motivation to continue an

Figure 183

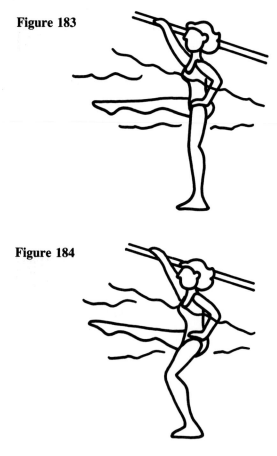

Figure 184

Leg Raise

exercise program diminishes as the back pain disappears. You know that stretching and strengthening is critical to your well-being. Perhaps going to a structured exercise class at least twice a week will help you stay on track.

If you consider joining a program or health club, request a complimentary visit to observe the procedures, equipment, and instructor attitude and rela-

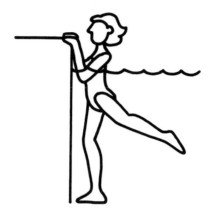

Figure 185
Extension Stretch

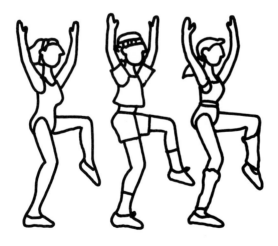

Figure 186
Exercise Class

tionships with students. Every exercise class should include a warm-up and cool-down period. Beginners should be shown how to modify activities so they can start the program slowly and build up tolerance to the exercises. Many classes do not have these protective factors, and newcomers to an exercise class can become candidates for a serious episode of back pain.

Many exercise instructors have had no formal training in exercise physiology or anatomy. They do not realize the potential for severe back injury if exercises are performed by individuals who are not physically able to comply with the routine. As the back owner, you will have to decide whether the exercise class and/or exercise program is appropriate for you.

You may feel comfortable performing only 85% of the exercises. In that case, don't worry about the other 15%. And don't be intimidated by the program or the instructor. You are the person who knows what you can and can't do...listen to your back!

RECREATIONAL ACTIVITIES

Although floor exercises are beneficial, the best type of physical activity is a recreational activity (preferably aerobic) that you enjoy and participate in on a regular basis. Recreational activities are healthy not only for your body, but also for your mind and emotions. The experts recommend at least 30 minutes of aerobic activity three times a week, and more if you can work it into your schedule. You don't need to excel or be a professional athlete to enjoy many activities. Give yourself a chance to get in shape, practice consistently, and

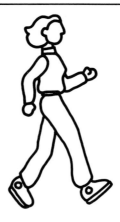

Figure 187
Fast Walking

you will improve no matter what activity you pursue. If you have been inactive for some time, set realistic goals for yourself. Don't get discouraged if you cannot perform as well as you think you should. Remember, anytime you suddenly increase your activity you will get sore. Keep exercising! You will work the soreness out as you increase your strength and flexibility. However, if soreness persists, you can use the first-aid techniques that are beneficial for muscle spasm. These are explained in Chapter 6; they are equally effective for muscle soreness.

Fast Walking (Figure 187)

This is our favorite exercise for easy conditioning and aerobic benefits. The only special equipment you need is a pair of good walking or jogging shoes that have crepe or rubber soles. Before you buy them, identify the surface on which you will be walking and inform the shoe salesman so he can select appropriate shoes for you to try on. If you are walking on a soft surface such as grass, you will need different footwear than if you are walking on pavement.

You can begin walking almost immediately after an episode of back pain. It is usually advisable, even while you have back pain, because it will keep you in good physical condition. You can also start a walking program after surgery, but check first with your doctor.

As a rule of thumb, a good pace is one mile in 15 minutes. The following chart will give you more specific guidance about pace and timing.

FAST WALKING EXERCISES

If you do	Start walking	Gradually progress to
Sedentary or light house/yard work	1/10 mile (about 2 city blocks)	1 mile in 20 min. 1 mile in 15 min.
Regular house/ yard work & light exercise	2/10 mile (about 4 city blocks)	1 mile in 18 min. 1 mile in 15 min.
Moderately heavy house/yard work & moderate/light exercise	3/10 mile (about 6 city blocks)	1 mile in 15 min.
Moderately heavy or heavy house/ yard work & occasional exercise	4/10 mile (about 8 city blocks)	1 mile in 15 min.
Heavy house/yard work & light exercise on a regular basis	1/2 mile (about 10 city blocks)	1 mile in 15 min. 2 mile in 30 min.

▼

If you live in a place with cold or wet weather, consider walking in shopping malls. Many of them open early in the morning and are staffed with security personnel so you can walk safely in a comfortable atmosphere. You can either time yourself and walk at your pace for 15 to 30 minutes, or find out if the mall management has marked off the distance from one store to another. It is an excellent way to window-shop. Take a friend, and it will be more fun.

It is very important to pace yourself when beginning a walking program. In order to attain a 15-minute mile, you must walk:

1/10 mile (2 blocks)	in	1 min., 30 sec.
2/10 mile (4 blocks)	in	3 min.
3/10 mile (6 blocks)	in	4 min., 30 sec.
4/10 mile (8 blocks)	in	6 min.
1/2 mile (10 blocks)	in	7 min., 30 sec.
6/10 mile (12 blocks)	in	9 min.
7/10 mile (14 blocks)	in	10 min., 30 sec.
8/10 mile (16 blocks)	in	12 min.
9/10 mile (18 blocks)	in	13 min., 30 sec.
1 mile	in	15 min.

Jogging (Figure 188)
Jogging puts more pressure on your discs than fast walking, but if you want to jog, we encourage you to do it as long as it does not make your back hurt too much. Stretching before you jog is critical to your back health. It is especially important to stretch your hamstring muscles before you start to run. If you have not run for a long time because of back pain, start slowly and alternate walking with running. You should be able to fast-walk five miles without any back pain before you begin a jogging program.

Bicycling (Figure 189)
This is one of the best recreational activities for excellent back and aerobic health. However, before you ride, check the angle of your bicycle seat to the

▼

handlebars. You may have to lower the seat and/or raise the bars. They should be positioned so you feel comfortable and your back doesn't hurt. Always stretch before you ride. Also, you will want to develop strong leg and thigh muscles, so concentrate on an exercise program that includes leg raises, partial squats, and others that are pertinent to this activity.

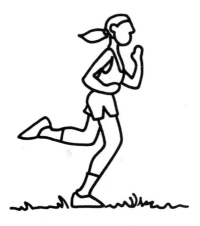

Figure 188
Jogging

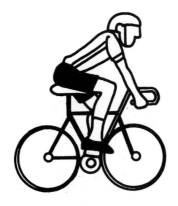

Figure 189
Bicycling

Tennis and Racquetball (Figures 190, 191, 192)
Both of these sports require dexterity and flexibility, and any sport that requires use of a racquet has the potential for twisting injuries. Therefore, you should concentrate on improving your body mechanics before you go back to playing. Find a friend who will let you take it easy for the first couple of weeks. Lob the ball while you are getting into condition. Keep your knees bent when you serve. Stay on your toes; keeping your body weight on the balls of your feet will lead to pivoting. Concentrate on pivoting.

Competition adds stress to your muscles, so warm up and cool down with stretching exercises. Tired muscles are most susceptible to injuries. Rest by walking around or lying down in the resting position. Try not to sit for long periods of time after a vigorous activity.

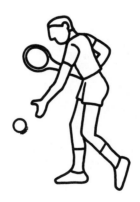

Figure 190
Tennis

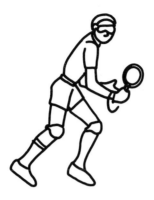

Figure 191
Racquetball

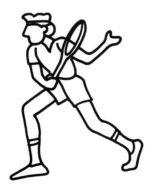

Figure 192
Pivoting

Golf (Figure 193)

Unfortunately, golf puts pressure on the lumbar discs because twisting is required as you take the clubhead back and drive it through the ball. However, unless you have had a severe problem, we encourage you to continue playing.

Stretching is mandatory! Start by practicing swinging your middle irons, and use them as you would a putter with a short arc. Concentrate on shifting your weight. You will reduce the twisting of your lumbar spine if you turn your toes out slightly and put your heels closer together. Cut your back swing to three-fourths of the length it was before you had back trouble, and try to pivot on the balls of your feet.

Bowling (Figures 194, 195)

Good body-mechanics techniques are tremendously helpful if bowling is your favorite pastime. You need strong thigh muscles to support your upper body and the weight of the bowling ball. Place a hand on your knee for additional support as you release the ball and it will increase your balance. Remember, if you are right-handed, the right side does all the twisting. Equalize the stress by warming up with the other hand holding the ball. You don't have to release the ball; just swing it on the opposite side to even out the pressure.

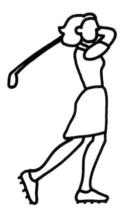

Figure 193
Golf

Baseball and Softball (Figure 196)
Anytime you use a piece of recreational equipment with a handle, you have a possibility of twisting your low back. Batting is no exception, because it requires twisting motion. Your best protection comes by warming up before you play and using the diagonal stance, which allows you to shift your weight as you swing the bat. It is also important to remember that strong quadriceps muscles and abdominal muscles help protect your back whether you are fielding, batting or running the bases.

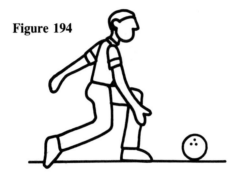

Figure 194

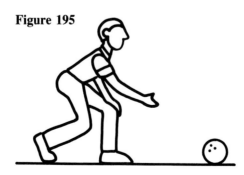

Figure 195

Bowling

Miscellaneous

There is an exercise category described as "other." Obviously a multitude of activities that are beneficial to your general health can be listed here. These may be non-sports activities, such as dancing, but they require some physical dexterity and physical demands. (Figure 197) As an example, dancing is good for you aerobically. If you are dancing regularly, you may be getting more of a workout than someone who plays softball. It is weight-bearing—which is particularly desirable if you are an osteoporosis candidate—and will help maintain the strength and flexibility that is so important to your healthy back.

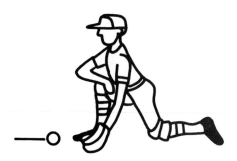

Figure 196
Baseball and Softball

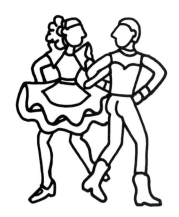

Figure 197
Dancing

If you are interested in joining a class, check with your local YMCA, or perhaps the parks and recreation department in your city. They will know what is available and the level of expertise required.

We have not covered all of the activities available, but hopefully we have touched on an activity that interests you. If not, the concepts you have learned remain the same no matter what activity you choose. Recreational activities are more than fun—they enhance your quality of life, contribute to your fitness, and provide a release for tension and stress. But you must begin any recreational situation using common sense, good body-mechanics techniques and lots of stretching. Start slowly and increase your endurance. If you are not comfortable with the activity you have chosen to pursue, take lessons so you can perform properly and with confidence. Above all, listen to your back!

▼

6

▼

Just In Case:

First Aid and Home Treatment

"**I** can't believe it is end of summer, and the cottage has to be closed up until Spring! What a job!" lamented Pam. "Terry and the kids have to take out the pier and the boat and put all of it in the garage. I guess I had better start clearing out all of the bedding and pack it in the truck. We should have started this project on Friday, but it was too pretty, and the fish fry was important to the kids. It is going to be a long time before we can do that again."

Allison and Josh went down to the dock to help their dad with the lakefront chores while Pam started cleaning and stripping beds. The furniture had to be covered with sheets, the rugs needed to be hung out and shaken, all of the food in the kitchen had to be packed in boxes for the winter or packed in the truck—and it had to be done by dark so they could get home. School started in the morning, and Pam wasn't sure whether Josh and Allison were ready with their supplies and books.

Both Pam and Terry spent the day pulling, pushing, lifting, packing, and finally left for home at about 5 p.m. Two hours and 100 miles later they pulled into the garage. Unfortunately, the boxes had to be labeled and put in the attic; then dinner had to be prepared and the kids had to be organized for school. Everyone finally fell into bed, exhausted, about midnight. The next morning Pam and Terry could hardly creep out of bed. They both had back pain. Terry's back pain was tolerable, but Pam could hardly struggle to the kitchen to fix breakfast.

"How in the world could this be happening to me?" she fretted. "I used good body mechanics all day, and I thought I was really careful. Now what do I do? I need help!"

▼

▼

Wayne looked in the mirror disapprovingly and chided himself. "You are going to be 40 years old next week, and you look like it! The extra 10 pounds is all in the middle, surrounded by sags. No more procrastination. You are heading to the track right now!"

And that is exactly what he did. Not only did he run a mile on Friday, Saturday, and Sunday, but he also played tennis every afternoon. He could almost feel himself returning to his former svelte self by the time Monday arrived. It was certainly not time to give up, so he ran every night after work, did a few sit-ups and lost three pounds the first week.

"This is a snap. I will be in fighting condition in a few more days," he crowed.

He upped his distance to two miles and added a few more rigorous floor exercises. Four days later, he felt the first stab of severe back pain.

"How in the world could this be happening? Just when I was getting into good shape. Now what do I do? I need help!"

Now that you are a back expert, you should be pain-free for the rest of your life, right? Although we would like to guarantee that, unfortunately, we cannot. Everyone forgets to use perfect body mechanics now and then, and the price for that is a backache. Also, degeneration continues as you age, so back pain becomes increasingly likely after everyday occurrences such as sitting for long periods, performing tasks too quickly, or playing golf without stretching adequately. Sometimes back pain occurs for no apparent reason. Therefore, you need to know first-aid techniques for those times.

First aid for back pain works well in most cases. Don't wait to see if it is going to disappear in a few days. Once the pain-spasm cycle gets started, it becomes difficult to break. Using proper first-aid techniques will allow you to continue with your activities.

SHOULD YOU REST?

Historically, the treatment for back pain was heat and bed rest. In one sense, that was logical; an injured area must have rest in order to repair itself. That is the reason a broken bone is immobilized in a cast. That is also the reason why doctors used to advise bed rest for extended periods following surgery. However, doctors have since learned that while surgical incisions healed nicely from such treatment, the rest of the body deteriorated rapidly. By the time patients recovered from surgery, they were almost too weak to stand up. If you have had surgery during the last decade, you know that now you are expected to be on your feet almost from the time you are out of the recovery room. The entire body functions better if all parts are kept moving.

▼

The same thing is true in relation to an episode of back pain. Assuming that a person is healthy at the onset of pain, statistics give that person a 90% chance that the back pain will disappear in two to six weeks. However, if that time is spent in bed, muscles in the rest of the body will atrophy or weaken because they are not being used.

The issue is how to rest the injured area to promote healing, while maintaining activity so the body doesn't lose function. The answer lies in the definition of rest. Rest is a state of inactivity, but it is not necessarily restricted to a bed. You can rest in a prone position using the body-mechanics techniques that are

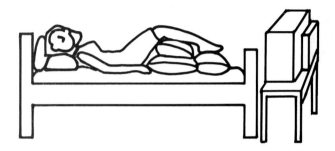

Figure 198
The resting position will reduce disc pressure when your back hurts.

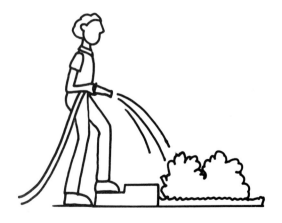

Figure 199
Rest your back by putting a foot up while you are working.

most comfortable. You can watch television by lying down on the floor with your feet on an ottoman or lying on the couch with a couple of pillows under your knees. (Figure 198) You can water the lawn while standing with your foot on a step. (Figure 199) Or, you can read in your favorite chair as long as you have your knees higher than your hips. All of these positions will rest your back and promote healing.

How much rest do you need? Not as much as you might think. You do not need to spend 24 hours a day in a prone position. Listen to your back. A few hours a day devoted to inactivity, in addition to your regular sleep time, should be sufficient. Activities that are done slowly and deliberately, using body mechanics positions that put minimal pressure on your low back, will usually not aggravate your pain.

HOW DO YOU MAINTAIN FUNCTION?

Sitting around watching television all day can hardly be construed as functioning very well. Boredom and muscle deterioration are likely to take place at about the same time. For each day that a person does not use a group of muscles, it will take four to seven days to rehabilitate those muscles. The weakening process happens very quickly!

Function is difficult if you are in a lot of pain. That's why first-aid techniques are so critical. If you know some easy and practical first aid for back pain, it will be much easier for you to regain function.

Because muscles are your body's protective mechanism, they provide the first response to a negative situation with your back. This response is to contract as fast as they can to let you know something is wrong. If you have ever had muscle cramps in your calves or feet, you know it is uncomfortable, to say the least. The back pain you have is very likely due to muscle cramps, muscle spasms or at least muscle involvement. (A muscle cramp is an intermittent contraction of a muscle. A muscle spasm is a sustained muscle contraction as a reaction to more severe injury.) For that reason, first aid for muscle spasm is the first step in regaining function.

FIRST AID IS SPELLED A-I-M

If you were to cut your finger, you would immediately wash it off and probably apply a bandage to stop the bleeding and keep out dirt. That is obviously first aid. If you were to sprain your ankle while playing tennis, you would probably wrap it in ice as quickly as possible to reduce swelling and minimize pain. In either of these situations, you would not wait a week or two to see if the injury would repair itself. But how many individuals do nothing about their back pain for several days or weeks with the hope that it will go away? Actually, first aid for back pain is just as important as first aid for any other kind of injury.

The first-aid technique that is most effective in reducing back pain and promoting function is a comprehensive approach called A-I-M. It is an acronym for *anti-inflammatory, ice massage* and *movement.* These are the components that reduce back pain and facilitate recovery.

Anti-inflammatory medication

Aspirin is a very effective anti-inflammatory drug, as is ibuprofen, which also is available now as an over-the-counter drug. An anti-inflammatory drug should be started, along with other first-aid measures, at the first sign of back pain. (Figures 200, 201) Muscles that are in spasm are irritated (inflamed), so an anti-inflammatory is appropriate medication. If a nerve is involved, it also will be inflamed, and aspirin or ibuprofen will decrease the inflammation.

Figure 200

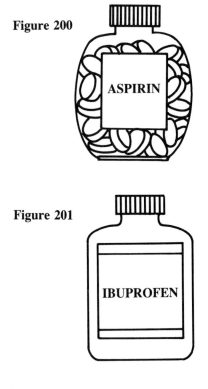

Figure 201

A-I-M.....The A is for Anti-inflammatory

Some people should not or cannot take aspirin. Most of these people already know who they are. In case you don't, check with your doctor before taking aspirin or ibuprofen if: you have any kind of bleeding problems such as stomach ulcers; you are allergic to aspirin; you have heart or circulatory problems; you are on other medication. However, *as long as they drink plenty of fluids,* most people can take two or three aspirins four times a day for several days while they are experiencing acute back pain. That means a big glass of water with each dose! If you have ringing in your ears at any time or an upset stomach, you need to quit taking those drugs immediately.

If you cannot tolerate aspirin or ibuprofen, you may take acetaminophen, an aspirin substitute. It does not have anti-inflammatory properties, so it will not be as effective in reducing inflammation as aspirin or ibuprofen products. However, it will at least decrease some of the pain.

The anti-inflammatory medication (or other pain reliever) should be taken for several days according to the schedule on the label so it has a chance to do what it is designed to do—reduce pain and decrease inflammation. It is important to keep the blood level of the anti-inflammatory high and constant for maximum effectiveness. If necessary, experiment with various products to see which one works best for you. If one product upsets your stomach, try another that has an antacid agent or a buffering agent. Some aspirin products contain caffeine and may keep you awake, some dissolve more quickly than others (lessening the chance of stomach irritation), and product strengths vary. Learning to read labels of over-the-counter drugs is important no matter what you are trying to treat.

Ice
The second part of the A-I-M plan is application of ice to the affected area. Ice massage is the kind of treatment that is more fun to give than to receive, but it is very effective in reducing pain and irritation in the low back and neck.

About now you are saying to yourself, "But I have this wonderful heating pad that I always use." However, heat increases circulation and ice decreases circulation. Heat increases swelling and ice decreases swelling. Increased circulation and swelling cause greater inflammation, with resulting discomfort, and may prolong healing. Ice also has a numbing effect so pain is decreased. With the decrease in pain, it is possible to stretch the muscles back to normalcy. Remember, muscles cannot stretch by themselves; they have to have assistance.

For these reasons, ice has become the "treatment of choice" during the last few years. Fortunately ice massage is not only easy to apply, but inexpensive and handy as well. To make an ice compress, simply freeze water in a paper or

▼

foam cup. Any size will do, but the size you use for coffee or a soft drink will work nicely. (Figure 202) The edge of the cup can then be peeled back a little to expose the ice, while the cup protects the hands of the person giving the ice massage. (Figure 203)

Ice massage is cold and messy, but so effective that it is worth the bother. If you can reach the injured area, you can apply the ice yourself—but it is more pleasant to have someone else apply it for you. If someone else is going to do it, lie down on the bed, couch or floor with a pillow under your abdomen.

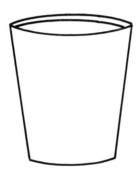

Figure 202
Freeze water in a paper or foam cup to make an ice cylinder for ice massage.

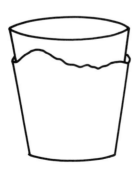

Figure 203
Tear off the top edge to expose the ice for ice massage.

▼

▼

Cover the pillow with a towel or two. The ice will melt quickly when in contact with warm skin, so you may need several towels to protect pillows, furniture or carpet.

Tear off the top couple of inches of the cup to expose the ice. The ice should be rubbed *gently* in a circular motion over the muscle spasm. (Figure 204) The ice massage should be applied a minimum of five minutes and a maximum of ten minutes. This should be timed. If the pain is only on one side of the spine, 5 to 7 minutes is appropriate. If the pain is on both sides of the spine, 7 to 10 minutes total time is appropriate. You can alternate 1 minute of ice massage on each side so that the entire area is adequately covered. Only the area over the muscle spasm—not directly over the spine—should be rubbed. The ice won't hurt the spine, but the backbone is very close to the skin surface and the rubbing won't be comfortable. It is important to time the ice massage. Frostbite can occur if the ice is left on the skin too long, so the *ice should never be applied directly to the skin for more than 10 minutes!*

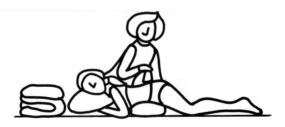

Figure 204
Gently rub the ice over the sore area for 5-7 minutes.

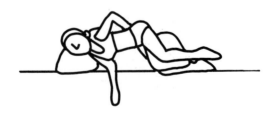

Figure 205
You can apply the ice yourself by lying on your side and reaching behind you.

▼

If you are going to apply the ice yourself, lie on your side (painful side up), with your knees drawn up, and reach behind you with the ice cup. (Figure 205) The most aggravating thing about this is the lack of sympathy from another person, and your arm will get tired—but don't give up. It is worth it.

You can also use an ice pack if you have one available and do not have an ice cup prepared. (Figure 206) However, the ice pack will not be as effective or provide relief as quickly. You should lie on your abdomen with a pillow underneath and place the ice pack on the muscle spasm for 20 minutes. The ice-pack wrapper or towel will protect you from frostbite. The ice pack is used for a longer period because it takes longer for the cold to penetrate to the muscle spasm.

Movement
The third part of the A-I-M treatment is movement or stretching. Once you have had ice massage, you will be numb. You can then stretch those tight muscles back to their normal range. To do so, *gently* bring one knee at a time toward your chin with your arms around your knee. (Figure 207) Don't use any jerking motions. Hold each knee for a count of 30. Do this exercise several times to stretch the back muscles.

If you prefer and it is comfortable, you can bring both knees up toward your chin at the same time. (Figure 208) A long stretch is better than a short stretch.

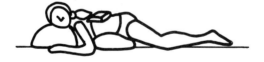

Figure 206
An ice pack over the muscle spasm will also give you relief.

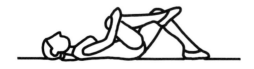

Figure 207
Gentle stretching will reduce the spasm once you have had ice massage.

You can do this movement as often as you like. Stretching helps the muscles relax.

Another stretch that you should find beneficial is the "hump and sag," (Figures 209, 210; see instructions on page 109). *If this stretch increases pain, don't do it.*

The best thing about A-I-M as a first-aid plan is that you can use ice massage and the stretches every couple of hours if you are in acute pain. It will break the pain-spasm cycle between the nerves and muscles by numbing the area and slowing down nerve impulses.

Figure 208

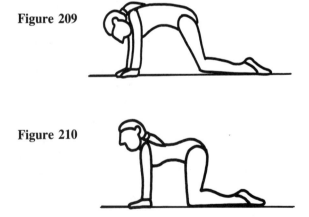

Bring both knees toward your chest slowly, and hold this position for the count of 30.

Figure 209

Figure 210

The hump-and-sag is an excellent stretching exercise. Arch your back like a mad cat, then sag like an old horse.

▼

Heat

Heat is certainly more "comforting" than ice. However, the maximum benefit from a heating pad occurs within 20 minutes or less. If you don't feel continued relief once you remove the heating pad, you might as well save the electricity and not bother. However, wet heat is a different thing. Many back-pain sufferers find that a warm shower or bath helps the muscles relax, and they can stretch the low-back muscles effectively afterward.

If you are really uncomfortable, you may want to try a combination of ice and heat. Use ice first for the numbing effect, stretch, and then get into a hot shower or a hot tub. Move slowly and deliberately while relaxing in warm water.

If you have frequent episodes of back pain and are considering buying a pool or spa, try a friend's first. See if it is beneficial for you before you invest in one. You own your back. Only you can know what works best for you.

SPECIAL TECHNIQUES FOR NECK PAIN

Although neck pain may be the result of overexertion or degeneration, it is more likely to be stress-induced or the product of poor body mechanics while sitting. Therefore, it is as important for you to develop body awareness about your upper spine as about your low back.

The same first-aid techniques—A-I-M—apply for neck pain as for back pain. You can use ice and stretching every couple of hours or as often as you deem necessary. Aspirin or ibuprofen is just as effective for neck pain as it is for back pain.

Ice can be applied in one of two ways. You can sit up in a straight-backed chair and have someone apply the ice or apply it yourself. (Figures 211, 212) Or, you can lie down in the same position you did for low-back pain and have someone apply the ice to your neck and shoulder region. (Figure 213) The amount of time you use the ice massage is exactly the same; five to ten minutes are appropriate. However, the stretching techniques are different.

In order to break the pain-spasm cycle of neck pain, you will want to stretch immediately after the ice application, just as you do for back pain. The following are range-of-motion exercises to increase your neck movement.

1. Gently move your head in a *"yes" motion*. Nod your head slowly, bringing your chin toward your chest. (Figure 214) Repeat five times.

2. *Saying "no"* will also stretch those stubborn, tight neck and shoulder muscles. Simply turn your head from side to side very slowly until you can turn enough to put your chin in line with your shoulder. (Figure 215) Repeat five times.

▼

Figure 211

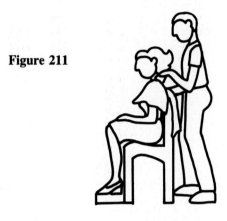

Figure 212

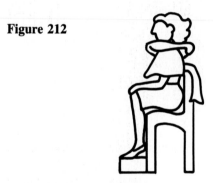

Figure 213

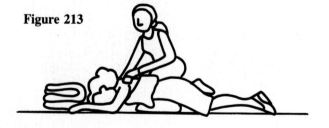

Ice massage is wonderful for stiff necks. Use the same technique that you did for low-back pain.

Figure 214
Saying "yes" helps stretch your neck muscles.

Figure 215
Saying "no" works for the same reason.

Figure 216
Using the "maybe" exercise will keep your neck muscles
flexible.

3. Now try *"maybe."* Tilt your head slowly from side to side. (Figure 216) Your ear should stay directly over your shoulder. Do this stretching exercise to increase flexibility in your neck muscles.

4. Once you have managed these three exercises, try some *shoulder rolls.* (Figure 217) Roll your shoulders forward, then backward in a circle. Do the exercise for 10-15 seconds to begin. Start with little circles and progress to large circles. This will relax your shoulder muscles as well as your neck muscles.

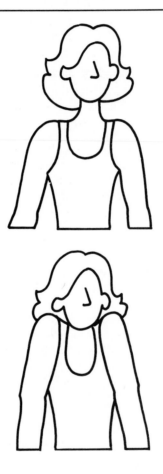

Figure 217
Shoulder rolls help mobilize stiff neck muscles.

DO'S AND DON'TS WHEN YOU ARE IN PAIN

When you are in pain, body mechanics becomes even more important. Using certain movements and positions will increase your function and hasten your recovery.

Sitting

Avoid sitting. If you must sit, get up and move around every 20 minutes. Don't sit without a good back support. Sitting with poor posture is certain to aggravate your back pain. Sit with your feet resting on something so your knees are higher than your hips. Also, use a small towel roll and small pillow behind your low back. This will help maintain the curve in your low back.

When standing up from a sitting position, move to the edge of your chair, position one foot in front of the other, and use your quadriceps muscles to stand. If the chair has arm supports, push off with your hands. To avoid leaning your upper body forward, keep your back straight.

Driving

Try to avoid driving. If you are a passenger, you can lie down in the back seat and bend your knees. If you must drive, move the seat close enough to the wheel so your knees are slightly higher than your hips. However, don't get so close to the wheel that you can't turn it. Use a towel roll or small pillow behind your low back and keep your chin pulled in. It is easy to become a head-thruster when driving.

Bending Forward

Try to avoid bending forward at the waist. This increases disc pressure. Kneeling to make beds and reach low levels is a good alternative.

Lying

A good firm support is desirable when lying down. The floor is too firm, a saggy mattress is too soft. Your mattress is fine if it is firm. When rising from a lying position, turn to one side, draw your knees up, and drop your feet over the edge. At the same time, push yourself up with your arms, and avoid bending forward at the waist.

Miscellaneous Tips

1. Change positions often. Do not stay in one place more than 30 minutes.

2. Stretch frequently. The more you stretch, the less likely the muscles will go into spasm. Stretching should be slow and deliberate.

▼

3. If you are not too uncomfortable, consider a walking program to increase your activity capabilities. If you are really uncomfortable, start with 1 block at a time, and increase your distance as your back will allow. This exercise can be ongoing and is beneficial for your entire spine.

4. Use common sense when you resume your normal activities. Do not overdo. You will regain function spontaneously if you use common sense and listen to your back!

WHEN TO SEE YOUR DOCTOR

If you have had a traumatic injury or are in severe pain, see your doctor immediately!

First aid is exactly that. It is the treatment plan to try first when you experience back pain. Now you are aware of good body-mechanics techniques, the most common reasons for back pain, and do's and don'ts to use at home and at work. However, this does not mean that you can always treat your own back without an expert. There are limits to self-help techniques.

Most back pain will disappear or subside in a few days with the use of anti-inflammatory medication, ice and/or heat, and appropriate stretching. If it does not, you should see your doctor.

Leg pain frequently occurs with an episode of back pain. It usually indicates some nerve involvement, but that may also subside after a few days of rest. If you have mild to moderate pain and you have tried all of the first-aid techniques for three to five days without improvement, you should call your physician.

However, don't call after office hours unless you have an emergency that requires immediate treatment. In that case, a trip to the emergency room is appropriate. Most mild pain can be managed until first thing in the morning, when you can call your doctor's office and schedule an appointment. An office visit is much less expensive than a trip to the emergency room.

Write down your concerns and questions *before* you see the doctor. Give him or her an accurate description of the episode that triggered pain and your response to it. Communication between you and your doctor is critical if both of you are to respond effectively to the situation. It will also help with your understanding of the treatment plan and tests that you will have.

So use first aid as it is intended: to give yourself an opportunity to heal and return to function as quickly as possible without expense. *Recognize your limitations* and seek expert advice when appropriate.

▼

CONTROLLING PAIN BY CONTROLLING STRESS

You know that tight tense muscles can result from stress. In fact, muscle spasms in your neck and back can occur as an aftermath of a back-pain episode. Once your muscles begin their "guarding" response, it is difficult to break the pain cycle. While A-I-M is usually beneficial, understanding methods of controlling stress will give you additional control over tense situations, thereby reducing muscle spasms associated with stress.

If you are going to control your mind and body, there are certain progressive steps you must learn and practice. This may sound simplistic, but it works. You can approach the problem in one of two ways. The first involves mental control, the second is conscious body control. Only you know which method will work best for you, but two components—isolation and concentration—are necessary with either approach.

First, plan on 20 minutes of isolation. Get comfortable, take the phone off the hook, lock the door, and turn off the television or radio. This part of the plan is essential for any kind of stress control.

Begin by focusing at a spot on the wall. Stare at this spot intensely, and put all other things out of your mind. Really concentrate on the spot.

When your eyes begin to feel tired, allow them to close on their own. Don't force them. After your eyes close, begin to think about your breathing. Take deep breaths from the bottom of your stomach. You will notice that your outgoing breaths remove tension from various parts of your body. Start thinking about *relaxing* your toes and work up to your shoulders. Then go back to your fingertips and focus on the different parts of your arm, working your way back to your shoulders. With each section of your body, concentrate on breathing and relaxing. You may feel warmth in each body part as you practice this technique; a relaxed state can raise your body temperature through improved blood circulation. Once you feel you have relaxed your entire body, open your eyes and see if you can maintain this state. It may take several months of practice before you have control over your body and environment at the same time.

If you find this method difficult, try *tightening* your entire body first. Close your eyes and concentrate on your tightened muscles. Then think about relaxing your toes, then your feet, your calves, your thighs—every part of your body up to your head. Concentrate on relaxing each tight muscle group. Do not relax the next part of your body until you are sure the part you are focusing on is very relaxed. For example, your toes and feet must be very

▼

relaxed before you can think about relaxing your calf muscles. Relax each small body section at a time. When you have reached your waist with this relaxation technique, concentrate on keeping your entire lower body relaxed for at least five minutes before you move on to the upper part of your body. You may need to especially focus on your back area and/or neck if you are currently experiencing pain.

These progressive relaxation techniques will give you better control over your body's response to your environment—and your comfort level. You should practice one of these techniques at least once a day, making this 20 minutes a top priority in your schedule. Not only can you reduce muscle spasm with these techniques, but you can also relax your mind and eliminate those sleepless nights when your mind is racing.

Mind control is like body-mechanics control. The change does not occur overnight. It takes a concentrated effort and continual practice before these lifestyle modifications become habit. However, once you establish these control techniques, they will be easy to use no matter where you are. We hope you will become "hooked" on these modifications.

WHAT NEXT?

Now that you have the basic information on HOW to take care of your back, are you going to do it? Or, are you going to make your doctor, your spouse and your employer responsible for the condition of your spine? Taking care of your spine, particularly your low back, is a 24-hour-a-day job. Changing your sitting, standing, lifting and sleeping habits is not easy. It would be wonderful if there were some magic pill that you could pop in your mouth once a day to cure back pain. Unfortunately, there isn't an easy solution. Taking care of your back is a challenge that requires a commitment to good body-mechanics techniques, stretching techniques, relaxation techniques—*everyday*.

How long will it take before these concepts become habits? It depends on your motivation. How much does your back hurt? Is it important to you to feel good? Do you care how you look? Is control of your back pain worth a little extra effort?

You did not develop back problems overnight, and you will not correct the problem in a day or two. The degenerative process continues, so don't expect miracles. Most of the people we work with say it takes four to six months of concentrated effort before these techniques become habit. However, the need to listen to your back, use proper body mechanics, and maintain physical fitness is never-ending. If you make up your mind that these things are important, and you really concentrate on changing the way you approach tasks, you can improve your quality of life in a very short time! Now it's up to you. ▼

▼

GLOSSARY

GLOSSARY

A

A-I-M—An acronym for first-aid treatment for back pain; it stands for anti-inflammatory, ice, and movement.

Anulus fibrosus—The tough outer layer of the intervertebral disc, which has a soft inner portion.

Arthritis—Inflammation of a joint; most arthritis is caused by degenerative changes related to aging.

B

Bar-resting position—A standing position using the diagonal stance, with one foot propped up.

Body mechanics—The body's posture or position and its relationship to activity or environment.

C

Cervical spine—The top portion of the spine (neck), composed of seven vertebrae.

Coccyx—The last four spinal vertebrae, which are attached to each other.

D

Degenerative disc disease—The daily wear and tear on the back, resulting in a narrowing of the discs.

Diagonal stance—A standing position in which one foot is placed in front of the other, providing a wide base of support and taking pressure off the lower back.

Discs—See *Intervertebral discs.*

F

Facet joints—The joints above and below each intervertebral disc, allowing the spine to bend.

I

Intervertebral discs—Oval structures that form the bending points between vertebrae and that function as "shock absorbers" to cushion the spine against force.

K

Kyphosis—An excess curvature of the thoracic spine called a "dowager's hump." This is a common occurrence in people with osteroporosis.

L

Lamina—The arch formed by the spinal vertebrae, protecting the spinal cord from exposure.

Ligaments—The strong bans that run from bone to bone giving stability to the spine during motion.

Lordosis—Excessive curvature of the low back, causing "sway back."

Lumbar spine—The lower spine, composed of 24 vertebrae that rest on a base formed by the sacrum and tailbone.

M

Muscle—The tissue that affects movement in each part of the body.

Muscle spasm—Strong, involuntary, painful contraction of muscles.

N

Nerve roots—Nerve projections from the spinal cord.

Nerves—The body's communication system; nerves carry messages back and forth between the brain and all body parts.

Nucleus pulposus—The soft pulp-like material inside the intervertebral disc.

O

Osteoporosis—A disease in which bones lose density, causing brittleness which leads to fractures.

P

Pivoting—A body-mechanics position to replace twisting, especially when moving a load; pivoting means moving shoulders, hips and feet in the same direction in which the load is being moved.

R

Rest—To put the body in a position that reduces the amount of pressure on the low back; does not mean bedrest.

S

Sacrum—Five attached vertebrae that form part of the base of the spine.

Sciatic nerve—Formed by multiple nerve roots from the lumbar spine; the sciatic nerve sends signals down the leg to control muscles and up the leg to provide sensations.

Scoliosis—A spinal abnormality known as "curvature of the spine."

Spina bifida—A congenital abnormality in which the arches fail to form over the spinal cord, leaving the cord unprotected.

Spinal stenosis—A narrowing of the spinal canal, which compresses the spinal cord and/or the nerve roots, cutting off their impulses to the muscles of the leg.

Spondylolisthesis—A spinal abnormality in which the fifth lumbar vertebra has a forward displacement upon the sacrum, or less commonly, the fourth lumbar vertebra is on the fifth lumbar vertebra.

T

Tailbone—See *Coccyx*.

Tendon—The fibrous tissue that attaches muscle to bone.

Thoracic spine—The middle part of the spine, composed of twelve vertebrae.

V

Vertebrae—Cylindrical segments of bone that form a column and link together to create the "scaffolding" of the spine.

INDEX

INDEX

A
A-I-M 140, 157
almost elbow touch 116
anatomical abnormalities 27
anti-inflammatory medication 141
anulus fibrosus 7, 157
applying makeup while sitting 57
arthritis 14, 157
aspirin 141

B
back pain without leg pain 104
bar-resting position 37, 38, 54, 57,
    66, 80, 157
baseball 133
basic body-mechanics principles
    101
bathing the baby or small child 58
bathroom activities, body mecha-
    nics 56
bed rest 138
bending forward when in pain 151
bicycling 128
body mechanics 31, 157
bowling 132

C
calf stretches 118, 120
carrying firewood 74
carrying groceries 51
carrying suitcases 88
carrying two small items 75
carrying two small suitcases 89
cervical spine 3, 6, 98, 157
changing your stance 79
chopping firewood 75
cleaning 63, 69
cleaning up with a push broom 69
climbing stairs and carrying a load
    82
coccyx 157
combination of ice and heat 147
competition 130
controlling pain by controlling
    stress 153

coughing and/or sneezing, body mechanics 93, 94

D
dancing 134
degenerative disc disease 157
diagonal stance 36, 43, 44, 46, 83, 87, 157
discs 7-9, 157
do's and don'ts when you are in pain 151
donkey kick 110
double knee-to-chest 106
drinking out of a bottle or can 101
driving or riding in the car, proper techniques 86, 151
dusting or cleaning at low levels 64

E
edging 70
emotional stress 14
exercise classes 124
exercises 104, 109
exercises after pain subsides 110
exercises as you increase your activity 118
exertion injuries 14
extension stretch 116, 124

F
facet joints 4, 7, 8, 157
fast walking 127
first aid 140, 152
flexibility 110
floor exercises 124

G
gardening 69
getting dressed, proper techniques 61
getting into and out of the car, proper techniques 86
getting up to your work level, proper techniques 56
golf 132

H
hamstring stretches 106, 108
handling loads 38

handling wet clothes 65
head-thrusting 95
health clubs 125
heat in treatment 138, 147
height of the computer screen 77
housekeeping activities 61
hump and sag 109

I
ibuprofen 141
ice compress 142
ice massage 141, 142, 148
ice pack 142
intervertebral discs 158
ironing 66, 67

J
jogging 128

K
keeping the load close 80
kitchen activities, body mechanics
    51
knees to chest 122
kyphosis 158

L
lamina 4, 158
laundry activities, body mechanics
    65
leg pain 152
leg raise 112, 123
leg-strengthening exercises 112
leisure activity, body mechanics 90
lifting, body mechanics 42
lifting a load from the floor to a
    table 81
lifting a small child out of the tub 59
lifting a small child out of a crib 60
lifting children out of the back seat
    86
lifting loads out of the back of the
    car 88
lifting objects out of the trunk 88
lifting something with a handle 82
lifting the trash basket 62
ligaments 10, 158
loading and unloading a dish-
    washer, proper techniques 55

lordosis 158
low-back stretch 106, 121
lumbar spine 3, 7, 158
lying when in pain 151
lying, body mechanics 40, 93

M
maintaining function 140
making your bed 60
manual material handling 81
miscellaneous tips 151
modified sit-up 104
movement in first aid 141, 142
moving material at waist height 81
moving material down from a high
  level 81
mowing the lawn 69
muscle spasm 19, 158
muscles 10, 158

N
neck positions, body mechanics 94
nerve root 10, 158
nerves 10, 158
nucleus pulposus 7, 158

0
obesity 20
osteoporosis 20, 158
overload 22

P
pain down your leg 109
partial squat 115
pelvic tilt 37, 104
pivoting 47, 48, 73, 74, 87, 130, 159
planting a garden or pulling up
  weeds 70
posture 24
predisposing condition 26
press-up 109
progressive quadriceps stretch 118
progressive relaxation techniques
  154
proper use of the telephone 101
pulling, proper techniques 85
pulling hoses 71-72

pushing and pulling, body mechanics 44, 84
pushing the lawnmower 68

R
racquetball 130
raking leaves 70
raking, proper techniques 71
range-of-motion exercises to increase your neck movement 147
reaching into cupboards 55
reading, body mechanics 91
reading or watching television in bed 91
recreational activities 126
rest 139, 159
resting position 41, 42, 90, 139
ruptured disc 28
ruptured or herniated disc 9

S
sacrum 3, 159
sciatic nerve 10, 159
scoliosis 26, 159
scrubbing the floor 64
shaving 99
shop or garage activities, body mechanics 67
shoulder hug 118
shoulder rolls 150
shoulder stretch 117
shoulder stretch and hug 116
shoulder-carry 81
shoveling 74
shoveling snow, proper techniques 74
sitting, body mechanics 32
sitting and eating 53
sitting at a drafting table 79
sitting at a typewriter 75
sitting at an assembly line 78
sitting at your desk 75
sitting hamstring stretch 108
sitting in an airplane seat 88
sitting in front of the television 90
sitting when in pain 151
sleeping activities, body mechanics 92

slouching 90
softball 133
special techniques for neck pain
147
spina bifida 27, 159
spinal stenosis 159
spondylolisthesis 27, 159
squat 42
standing, body mechanics 35
standing at the kitchen sink 54
standing for long periods 80
standing hamstring stretch 108
standing jobs 67
straight-leg raise 112
stretching 116
stretching exercise 146
stretching once you have had ice
massage 142
stretching your neck muscles 149
sweeping 61, 62

T
tailbone (coccyx) 3, 159
taking out the trash 61
telephone receiver, how to hold
101
tendon 159
tennis 130
thigh stretch 121
thoracic spine 3, 7, 159
three-point contact 82
transferring items into or out of the
refrigerator 52
transporting wet or dry clothes 67
traumatic occurrences 27
travel activities, body mechanics 86
trimming trees 71
trip to the emergency room 152
turtle position 96
twisting 47, 48, 72, 85, 87

U
using a computer terminal 77

V
vacuuming 62-63
vertebrae 3, 159

W
wall slide 114
watching television 90
water exercises 122
when you see your doctor 152
working in your shop or at a work
    bench 67
working on the car 67
workplace activities 75

NOTES

NOTES

NOTES